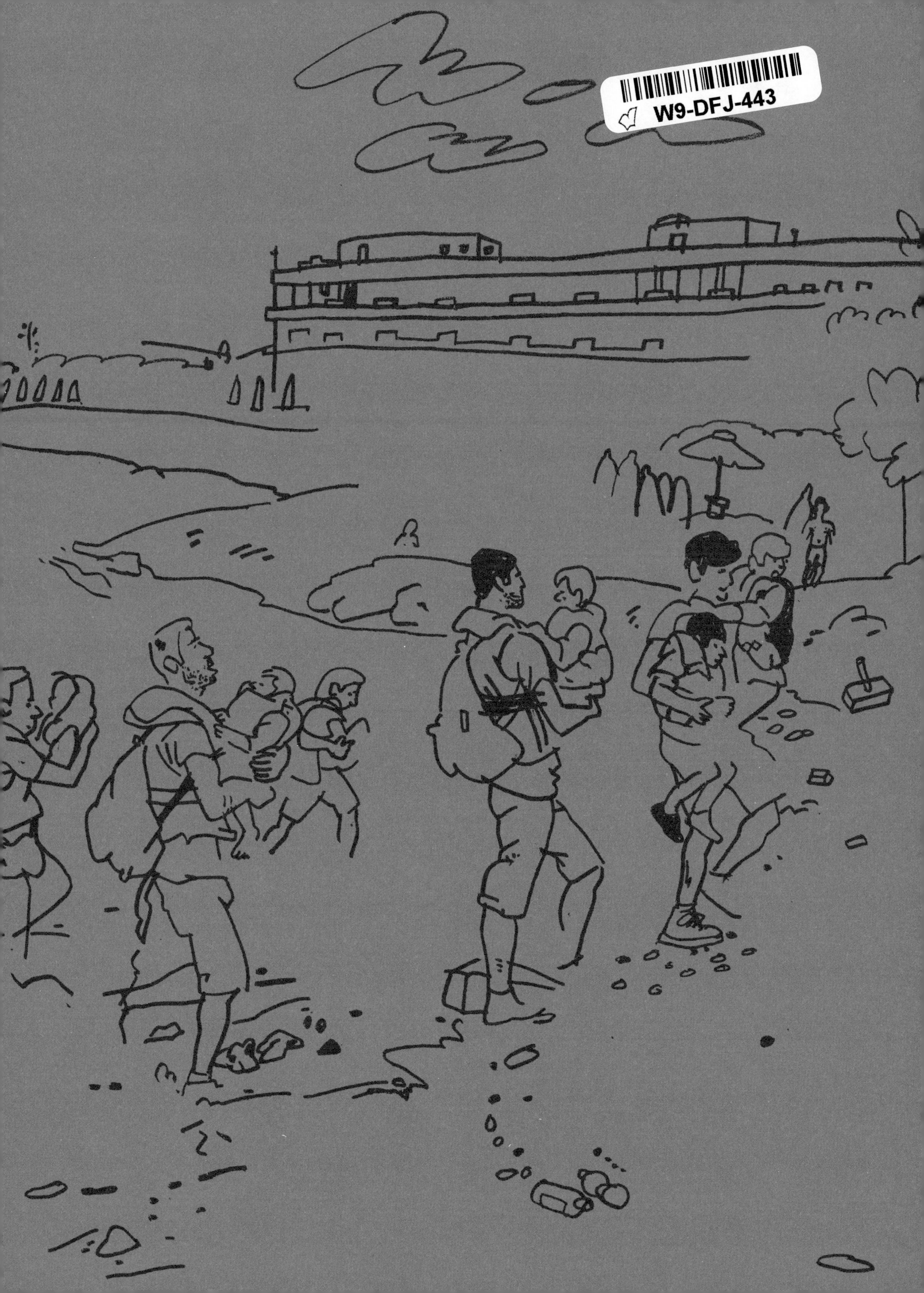

ESCAPING WARS AND WAVES

ENCOUNTERS WITH SYRIAN REFUGEES

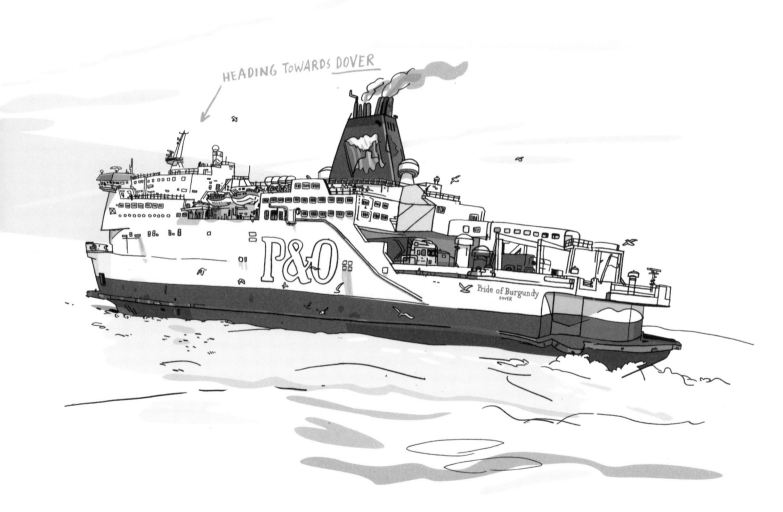

HEADING TOWARDS DOVER

P&O

Pride of Burgundy
DOVER

DRAWN & RECORDED BY OLIVIER KUGLER

THE PENNSYLVANIA STATE UNIVERSITY PRESS

UNIVERSITY PARK, PENNSYLVANIA

"BY NOW,
ALL THE SURVIVORS, ALL WHO AVOIDED HEADLONG DEATH
WERE SAFE AT HOME, ESCAPED THE WARS AND WAVES."

FROM THE ODYSSEY BY HOMER, TRANSLATION © ROBERT FAGLES, 1996

CATALOGING-IN-PUBLICATION DATA IS ON FILE WITH THE LIBRARY OF CONGRESS.

FIRST PUBLISHED BY EDITION MODERNE AS DEM KRIEG ENTRONNEN
COPYRIGHT © 2017 EDITION MODERNE, ZURICH, SWITZERLAND AND OLIVIER KUGLER
ALL RIGHTS RESERVED.
THIS EDITION COPYRIGHT © OLIVIER KUGLER 2018
PUBLISHED BY THE PENNSYLVANIA STATE UNIVERSITY PRESS,
UNIVERSITY PARK, PA 16802-1003
FIRST PUBLISHED IN ENGLISH BY MYRIAD EDITIONS, WWW.MYRIADEDITIONS.COM

THE PENNSYLVANIA STATE UNIVERSITY PRESS IS A MEMBER OF THE ASSOCIATION OF
AMERICAN UNIVERSITY PRESSES.

IT IS THE POLICY OF THE PENNSYLVANIA STATE UNIVERSITY PRESS TO USE ACID-FREE PAPER.
PUBLICATIONS ON UNCOATED STOCK SATISFY THE MINIMUM REQUIREMENTS OF AMERICAN
NATIONAL STANDARD FOR INFORMATION SCIENCES - PERMANENCE OF PAPER FOR PRINTED
LIBRARY MATERIAL, ANSI Z 39.48-1992.

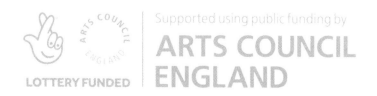
Supported using public funding by
ARTS COUNCIL
ENGLAND

"HELLO, MY NAME IS OLIVIER KUGLER, I AM A GERMAN REPORTAGE ILLUSTRATOR BASED IN LONDON. MÉDECINS SANS FRONTIÈRES COMMISSIONED ME TO PORTRAY SYRIAN REFUGEES, IN ORDER TO HELP RAISE AWARENESS ABOUT THEIR SITUATION. MAY I INTERVIEW AND TAKE PHOTOS OF YOU? THE PHOTOS WON'T BE PUBLISHED, BUT I NEED THEM AS REFERENCE FOR MY DRAWINGS." These were the words I used to introduce myself to Syrian refugees I met in Iraqi Kurdistan, Greece and France. Based on these encounters, which took place between 2013 and 2017, I created the drawings and texts which are collected in this book.

In December 2013 I travelled together with Julien Rey from Médecins sans Frontières (MSF) to Domiz Refugee camp. Accompanied by two Syrian Kurds, Mazen and Amer, who helped us with translations, we met open-hearted people who invited us into their tents and houses where they told us over a cup of tea about their lives back home, their escape from Syria and about the living conditions in the camp. Not all of the people I interviewed, or wanted to interview, were happy about the idea that their portraits would be published. Some were afraid that their relatives back in Syria, or they themselves, could get into trouble with one of the many warring factions in the conflict... or even with the authorities in the camp. There were also problems with my attempts to interview and photograph women. I would have loved to have depicted the busy goings-on inside one of the camp's beauty parlors, the young women putting on makeup and getting their hair done ahead of a wedding party, or the chain-smoking old lady who worked as a midwife... unfortunately, all my requests were turned down.

In the beginning of July 2015, I was asked by MSF if I would like to visit the Greek island of Kos to report on the stranded refugees. During my stay there, I frequently cycled out to the beaches, where, in the early morning, people arrived in overcrowded rubber dinghies. After they got themselves registered, they were told that they weren't allowed to board the next ferry to Athens. Instead they would have to wait, sometimes for weeks, for the documents that would give them permission to continue their journeys to Northern Europe. The local authorities provided neither accommodation nor showers or toilets for the refugees; many of them were sent to a dilapidated and already over-crowded hotel on the outskirts of the town, where a small MSF team looked after them. Other than in Domiz I found it relatively easy to get permission from women to take their pictures while they told me their stories. Nevertheless, I noticed that they weren't very comfortable with it —who would want to be photographed by a complete stranger in such a situation? But it was important to me that their voices should be heard, that they could share their stories, their frustration and their anger over the lack of support from the Greek authorities. One lady told me:

"IN EUROPE, I HAD HOPED, WE WOULD GET TREATED WITH RESPECT."

In 2016, during the Easter holidays, I took the ferry to Calais where I spent three days in the migrant camp, known as 'The Jungle.' Compared to Domiz and Kos, I found it even more difficult to meet people who were happy with me interviewing and photographing them. The camp at this time, was in the focus of the media. Perhaps many of the refugees became irritated with all the cameras being constantly pointed at them. Luckily, a member of the local MSF team helped me talk with some of the camp's residents.

In London, my studio is located in the same building as the Woman's Refugee Association. I told them about my work and they introduced me to Dr. Wafaa from Damascus, who attended their English language lessons.

Counterpoints Arts, an organization that supports art projects made by and about refugees, helped me to get a grant from the Arts Council England, which allowed me to work on this book. It was in the Counterpoints Arts office that I spotted the photo of a smiling boy with dark curly hair. It was Mohamad: he and his family had found refuge in Birmingham, where I visited them in October 2016.

Just after Christmas 2016, I spent some days at my parents' house. They introduced me to a family who had to leave their home in Deir-ez-Zor, Syria, and —for the time being—are now living in Simmozheim, in the Black Forest, the village where I grew up.

I am very grateful that I had the chance to meet the people I portrayed in my drawings. I feel connected to them and want to thank them very much for their patience and trust. I hope that their circumstances have improved significantly and wish them, and their compatriots, all the best!

KURDISTAN REGION

(IRAQ)

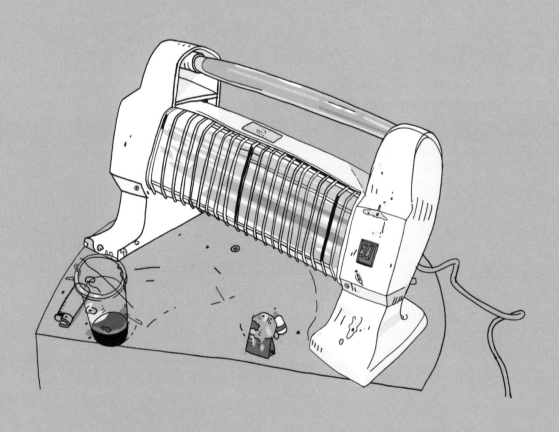

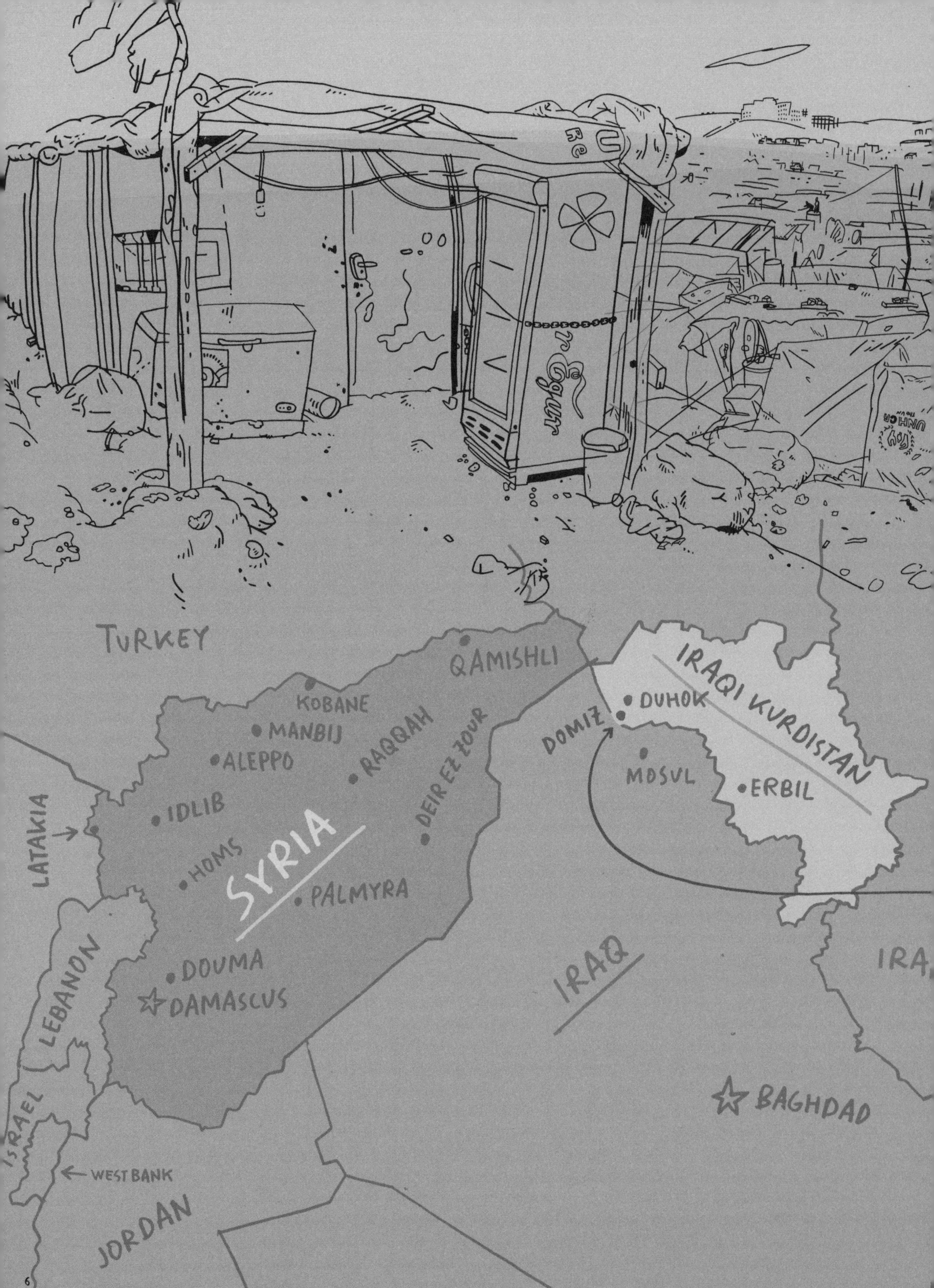
TURKEY
QAMISHLI
KOBANE
MANBIJ
ALEPPO
RAQQAH
DEIR EZ ZOUR
LATAKIA
IDLIB
HOMS
SYRIA
PALMYRA
DOUMA
DAMASCUS
LEBANON
ISRAEL
WEST BANK
JORDAN
IRAQI KURDISTAN
DUHOK
DOMIZ
MOSUL
ERBIL
IRAQ
BAGHDAD

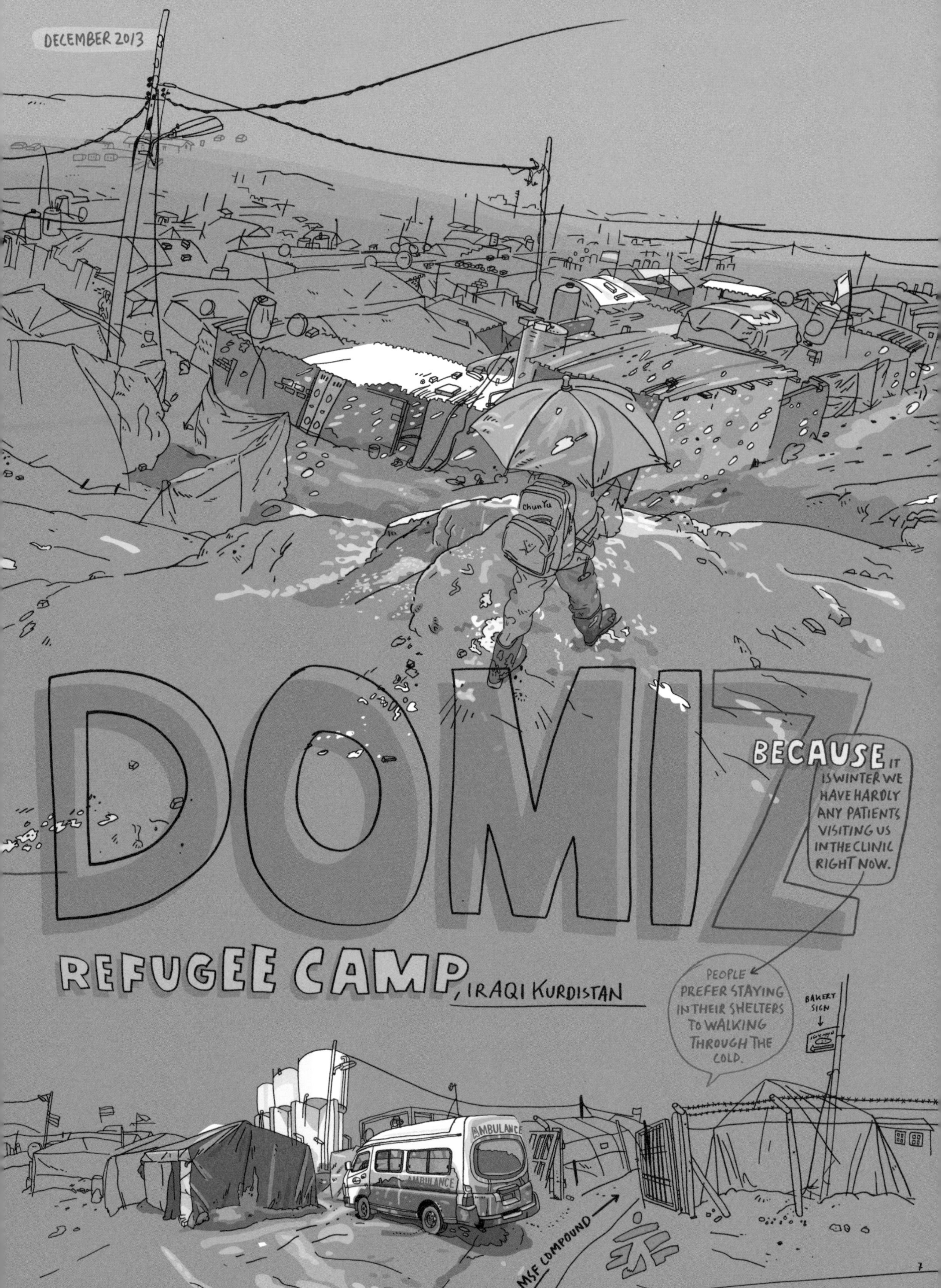
DECEMBER 2013
ChunYu
DOMIZ
REFUGEE CAMP, IRAQI KURDISTAN
BECAUSE IT IS WINTER WE HAVE HARDLY ANY PATIENTS VISITING US IN THE CLINIC RIGHT NOW.
PEOPLE PREFER STAYING IN THEIR SHELTERS TO WALKING THROUGH THE COLD.
BAKERY SIGN
AMBULANCE
AMBULANCE
MSF COMPOUND

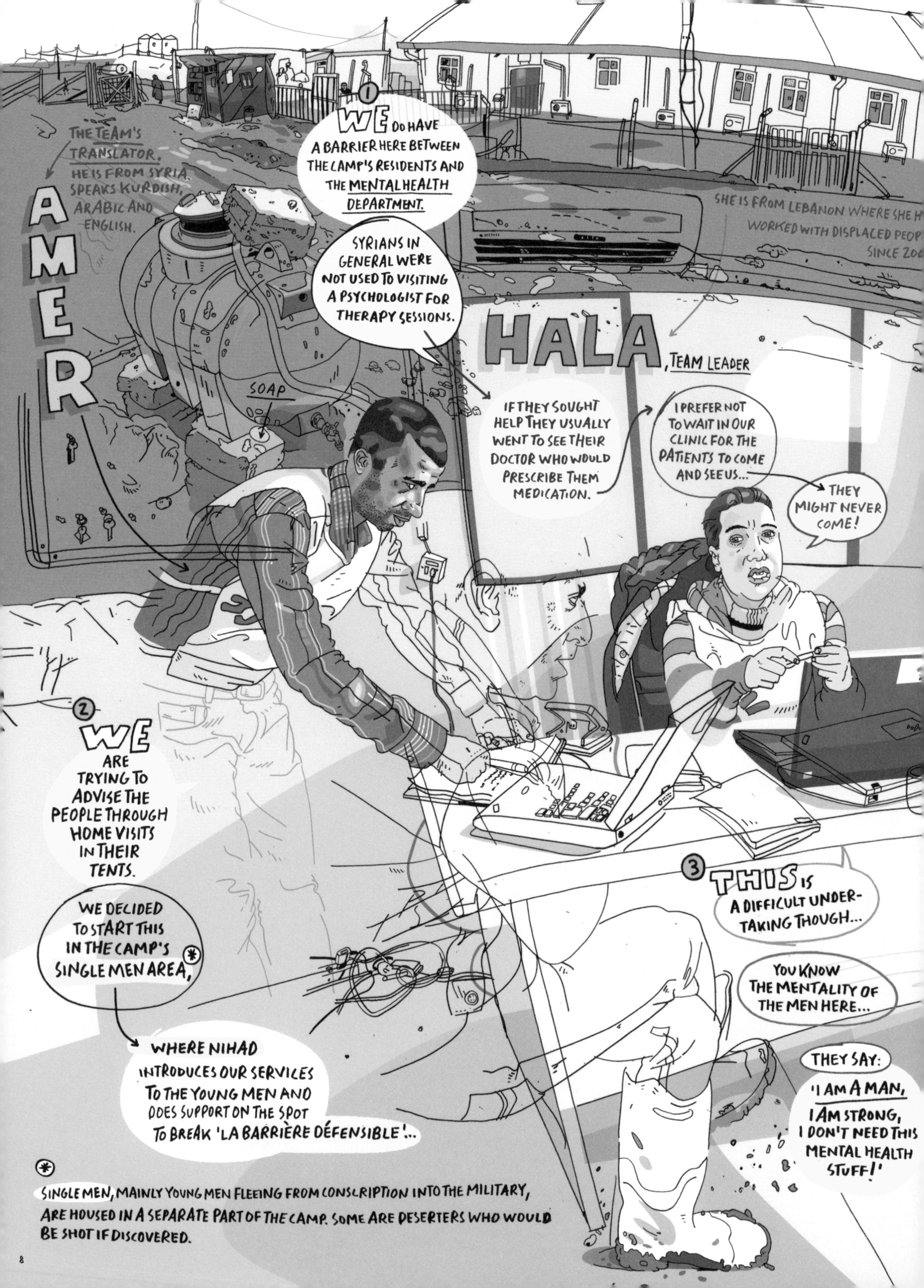

THE TEAM'S TRANSLATOR. HE IS FROM SYRIA. SPEAKS KURDISH, ARABIC AND ENGLISH.
AMER
① WE DO HAVE A BARRIER HERE BETWEEN THE CAMP'S RESIDENTS AND THE MENTAL HEALTH DEPARTMENT.
SYRIANS IN GENERAL WERE NOT USED TO VISITING A PSYCHOLOGIST FOR THERAPY SESSIONS.
SHE IS FROM LEBANON WHERE SHE H
WORKED WITH DISPLACED PEOP
SINCE 20
HALA, TEAM LEADER
SOAP
IF THEY SOUGHT HELP THEY USUALLY WENT TO SEE THEIR DOCTOR WHO WOULD PRESCRIBE THEM MEDICATION.
I PREFER NOT TO WAIT IN OUR CLINIC FOR THE PATIENTS TO COME AND SEE US...
THEY MIGHT NEVER COME!
② WE ARE TRYING TO ADVISE THE PEOPLE THROUGH HOME VISITS IN THEIR TENTS.
WE DECIDED TO START THIS IN THE CAMP'S SINGLE MEN AREA, (*)
WHERE NIHAD INTRODUCES OUR SERVICES TO THE YOUNG MEN AND DOES SUPPORT ON THE SPOT TO BREAK 'LA BARRIÈRE DÉFENSIBLE'...
③ THIS IS A DIFFICULT UNDERTAKING THOUGH...
YOU KNOW THE MENTALITY OF THE MEN HERE...
THEY SAY:
'I AM A MAN, I AM STRONG, I DON'T NEED THIS MENTAL HEALTH STUFF!'
(*)
SINGLE MEN, MAINLY YOUNG MEN FLEEING FROM CONSCRIPTION INTO THE MILITARY, ARE HOUSED IN A SEPARATE PART OF THE CAMP. SOME ARE DESERTERS WHO WOULD BE SHOT IF DISCOVERED.

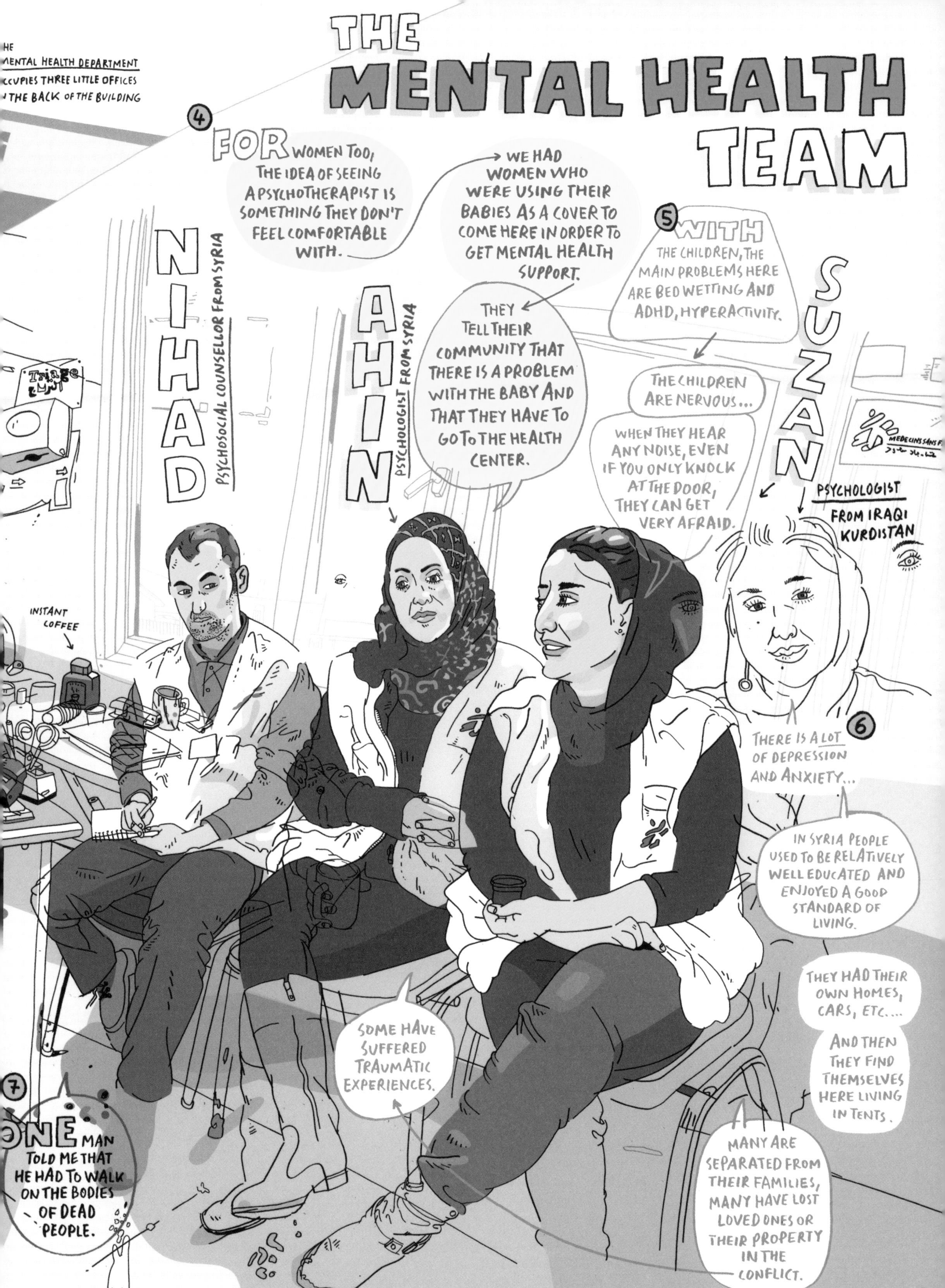

HE
MENTAL HEALTH DEPARTMENT
CCUPIES THREE LITTLE OFFICES
N THE BACK OF THE BUILDING
THE MENTAL HEALTH TEAM
4
FOR WOMEN TOO, THE IDEA OF SEEING A PSYCHOTHERAPIST IS SOMETHING THEY DON'T FEEL COMFORTABLE WITH.
WE HAD WOMEN WHO WERE USING THEIR BABIES AS A COVER TO COME HERE IN ORDER TO GET MENTAL HEALTH SUPPORT.
THEY TELL THEIR COMMUNITY THAT THERE IS A PROBLEM WITH THE BABY AND THAT THEY HAVE TO GO TO THE HEALTH CENTER.
NIHAD
PSYCHOSOCIAL COUNSELLOR FROM SYRIA
AHIN
PSYCHOLOGIST FROM SYRIA
5
WITH THE CHILDREN, THE MAIN PROBLEMS HERE ARE BED WETTING AND ADHD, HYPERACTIVITY.
THE CHILDREN ARE NERVOUS...
WHEN THEY HEAR ANY NOISE, EVEN IF YOU ONLY KNOCK AT THE DOOR, THEY CAN GET VERY AFRAID.
SUZAN
PSYCHOLOGIST FROM IRAQI KURDISTAN
Triage
INSTANT COFFEE
6
THERE IS A LOT OF DEPRESSION AND ANXIETY...
IN SYRIA PEOPLE USED TO BE RELATIVELY WELL EDUCATED AND ENJOYED A GOOD STANDARD OF LIVING.
THEY HAD THEIR OWN HOMES, CARS, ETC....
AND THEN THEY FIND THEMSELVES HERE LIVING IN TENTS.
7
ONE MAN TOLD ME THAT HE HAD TO WALK ON THE BODIES OF DEAD PEOPLE.
SOME HAVE SUFFERED TRAUMATIC EXPERIENCES.
MANY ARE SEPARATED FROM THEIR FAMILIES, MANY HAVE LOST LOVED ONES OR THEIR PROPERTY IN THE CONFLICT.

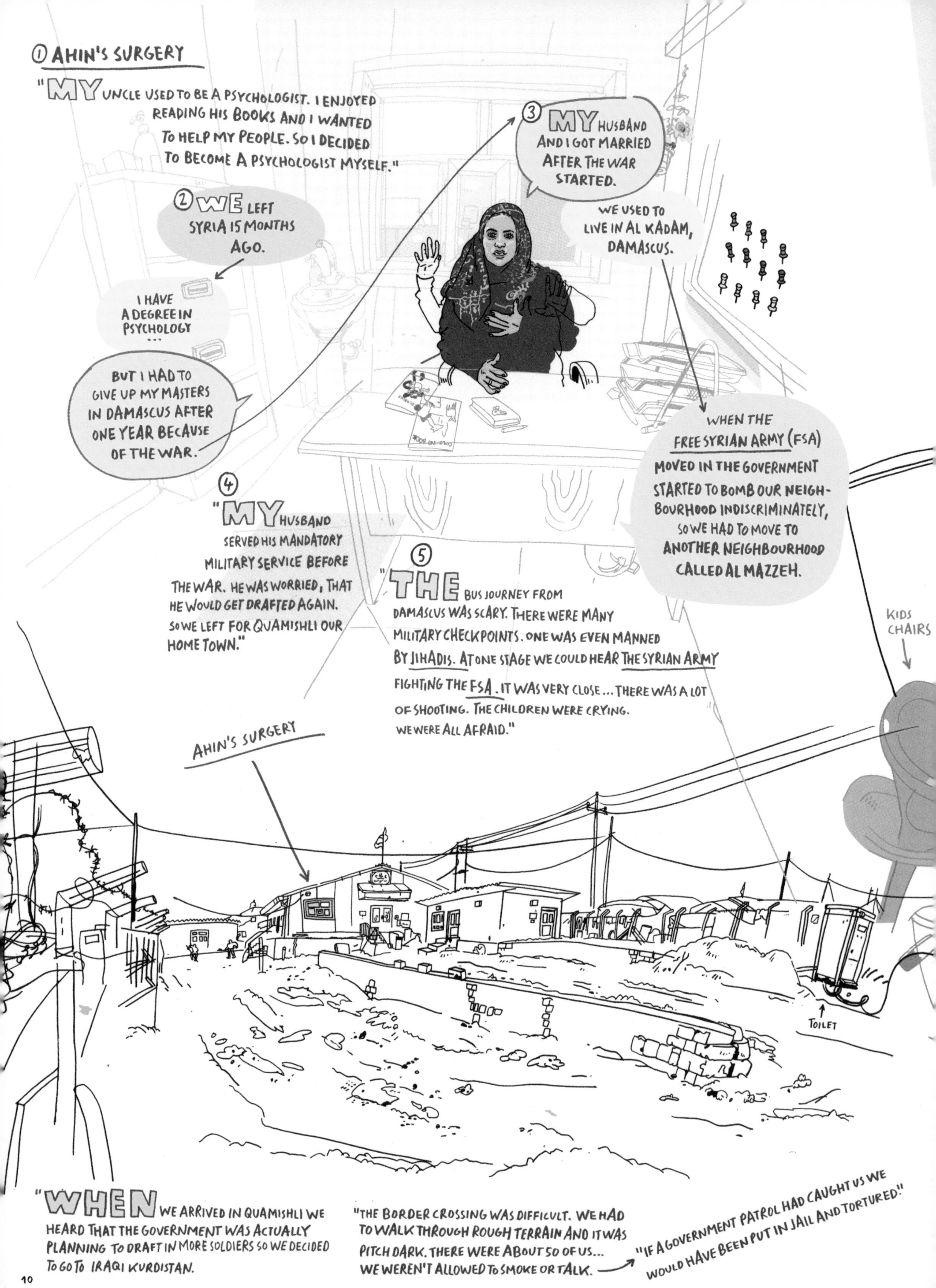
① AHIN'S SURGERY
"MY UNCLE USED TO BE A PSYCHOLOGIST. I ENJOYED READING HIS BOOKS AND I WANTED TO HELP MY PEOPLE. SO I DECIDED TO BECOME A PSYCHOLOGIST MYSELF."
② WE LEFT SYRIA 15 MONTHS AGO.
I HAVE A DEGREE IN PSYCHOLOGY ...
BUT I HAD TO GIVE UP MY MASTERS IN DAMASCUS AFTER ONE YEAR BECAUSE OF THE WAR.
③ MY HUSBAND AND I GOT MARRIED AFTER THE WAR STARTED.
WE USED TO LIVE IN AL KADAM, DAMASCUS.
WHEN THE FREE SYRIAN ARMY (FSA) MOVED IN THE GOVERNMENT STARTED TO BOMB OUR NEIGHBOURHOOD INDISCRIMINATELY, SO WE HAD TO MOVE TO ANOTHER NEIGHBOURHOOD CALLED AL MAZZEH.
④ "MY HUSBAND SERVED HIS MANDATORY MILITARY SERVICE BEFORE THE WAR. HE WAS WORRIED, THAT HE WOULD GET DRAFTED AGAIN. SO WE LEFT FOR QUAMISHLI OUR HOME TOWN."
⑤ "THE BUS JOURNEY FROM DAMASCUS WAS SCARY. THERE WERE MANY MILITARY CHECKPOINTS. ONE WAS EVEN MANNED BY JIHADIS. AT ONE STAGE WE COULD HEAR THE SYRIAN ARMY FIGHTING THE FSA. IT WAS VERY CLOSE... THERE WAS A LOT OF SHOOTING. THE CHILDREN WERE CRYING. WE WERE ALL AFRAID."
KIDS CHAIRS
AHIN'S SURGERY
TOILET
"WHEN WE ARRIVED IN QUAMISHLI WE HEARD THAT THE GOVERNMENT WAS ACTUALLY PLANNING TO DRAFT IN MORE SOLDIERS SO WE DECIDED TO GO TO IRAQI KURDISTAN.
"THE BORDER CROSSING WAS DIFFICULT. WE HAD TO WALK THROUGH ROUGH TERRAIN AND IT WAS PITCH DARK. THERE WERE ABOUT 50 OF US... WE WEREN'T ALLOWED TO SMOKE OR TALK.
"IF A GOVERNMENT PATROL HAD CAUGHT US WE WOULD HAVE BEEN PUT IN JAIL AND TORTURED."

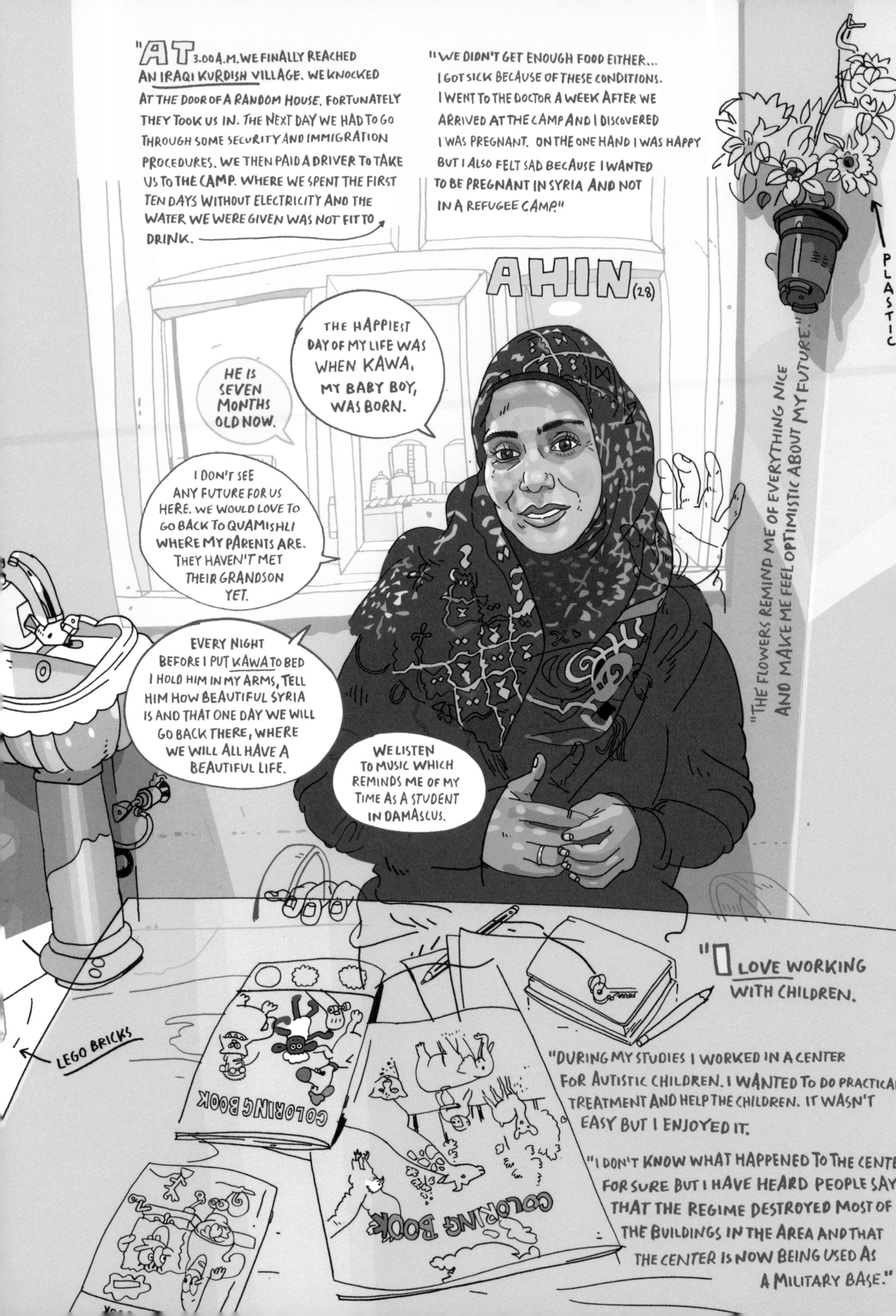
"AT 3.00 A.M. WE FINALLY REACHED AN IRAQI KURDISH VILLAGE. WE KNOCKED AT THE DOOR OF A RANDOM HOUSE. FORTUNATELY THEY TOOK US IN. THE NEXT DAY WE HAD TO GO THROUGH SOME SECURITY AND IMMIGRATION PROCEDURES. WE THEN PAID A DRIVER TO TAKE US TO THE CAMP. WHERE WE SPENT THE FIRST TEN DAYS WITHOUT ELECTRICITY AND THE WATER WE WERE GIVEN WAS NOT FIT TO DRINK.
"WE DIDN'T GET ENOUGH FOOD EITHER... I GOT SICK BECAUSE OF THESE CONDITIONS. I WENT TO THE DOCTOR A WEEK AFTER WE ARRIVED AT THE CAMP AND I DISCOVERED I WAS PREGNANT. ON THE ONE HAND I WAS HAPPY BUT I ALSO FELT SAD BECAUSE I WANTED TO BE PREGNANT IN SYRIA AND NOT IN A REFUGEE CAMP."
AHIN (28)
THE HAPPIEST DAY OF MY LIFE WAS WHEN KAWA, MY BABY BOY, WAS BORN.
HE IS SEVEN MONTHS OLD NOW.
I DON'T SEE ANY FUTURE FOR US HERE. WE WOULD LOVE TO GO BACK TO QUAMISHLI WHERE MY PARENTS ARE. THEY HAVEN'T MET THEIR GRANDSON YET.
EVERY NIGHT BEFORE I PUT KAWA TO BED I HOLD HIM IN MY ARMS, TELL HIM HOW BEAUTIFUL SYRIA IS AND THAT ONE DAY WE WILL GO BACK THERE, WHERE WE WILL ALL HAVE A BEAUTIFUL LIFE.
WE LISTEN TO MUSIC WHICH REMINDS ME OF MY TIME AS A STUDENT IN DAMASCUS.
PLASTIC
"THE FLOWERS REMIND ME OF EVERYTHING NICE AND MAKE ME FEEL OPTIMISTIC ABOUT MY FUTURE."
LEGO BRICKS
COLORING BOOK
COLORING BOOK
"I LOVE WORKING WITH CHILDREN.
"DURING MY STUDIES I WORKED IN A CENTER FOR AUTISTIC CHILDREN. I WANTED TO DO PRACTICAL TREATMENT AND HELP THE CHILDREN. IT WASN'T EASY BUT I ENJOYED IT.
"I DON'T KNOW WHAT HAPPENED TO THE CENTER FOR SURE BUT I HAVE HEARD PEOPLE SAY THAT THE REGIME DESTROYED MOST OF THE BUILDINGS IN THE AREA AND THAT THE CENTER IS NOW BEING USED AS A MILITARY BASE."

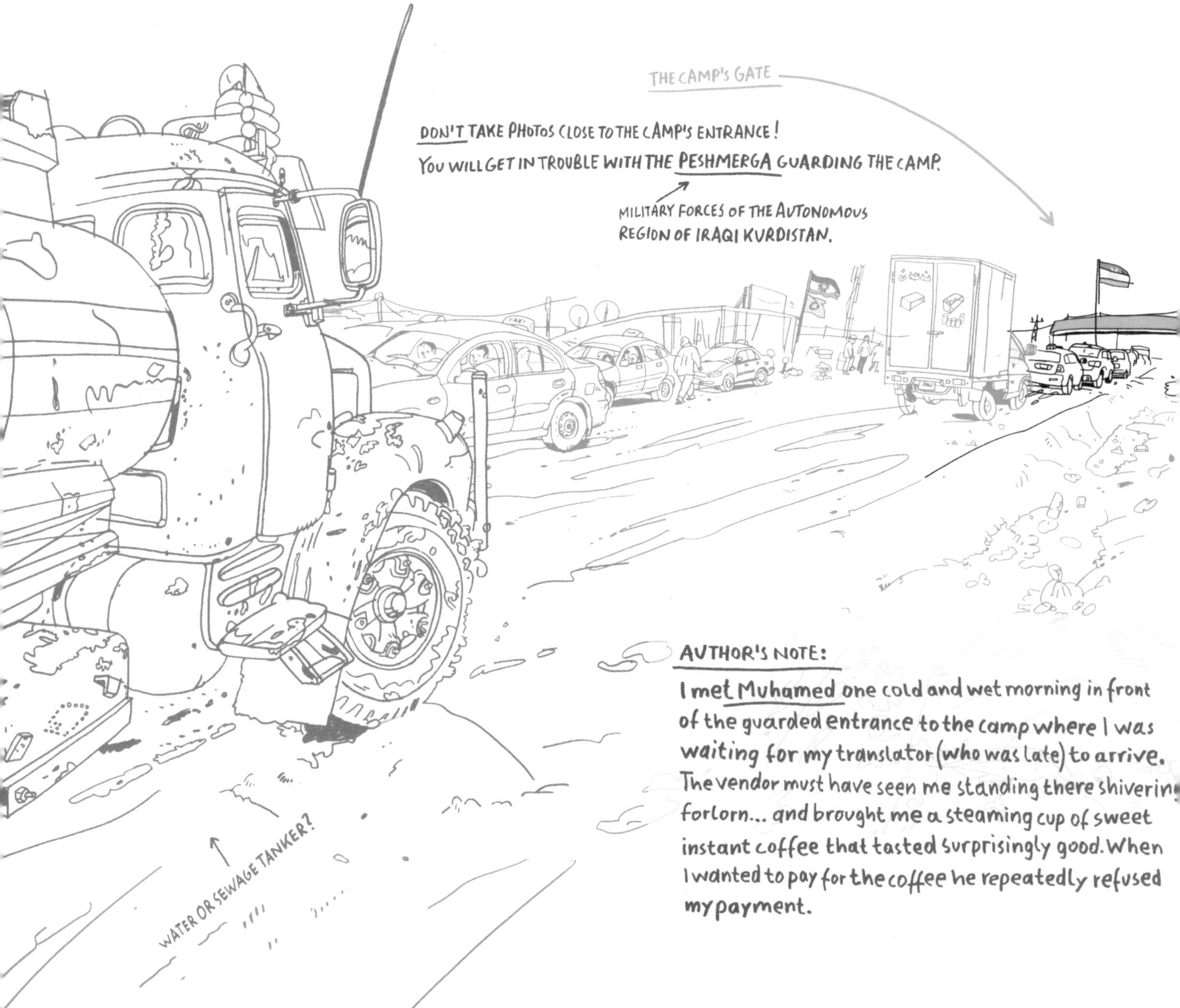
THE CAMP's GATE
DON'T TAKE PHOTOS CLOSE TO THE CAMP's ENTRANCE!
YOU WILL GET IN TROUBLE WITH THE PESHMERGA GUARDING THE CAMP.
MILITARY FORCES OF THE AUTONOMOUS REGION OF IRAQI KURDISTAN.
WATER OR SEWAGE TANKER?

AUTHOR'S NOTE:

I met Muhamed one cold and wet morning in front of the guarded entrance to the camp where I was waiting for my translator (who was late) to arrive. The vendor must have seen me standing there shivering forlorn... and brought me a steaming cup of sweet instant coffee that tasted surprisingly good. When I wanted to pay for the coffee he repeatedly refused my payment.

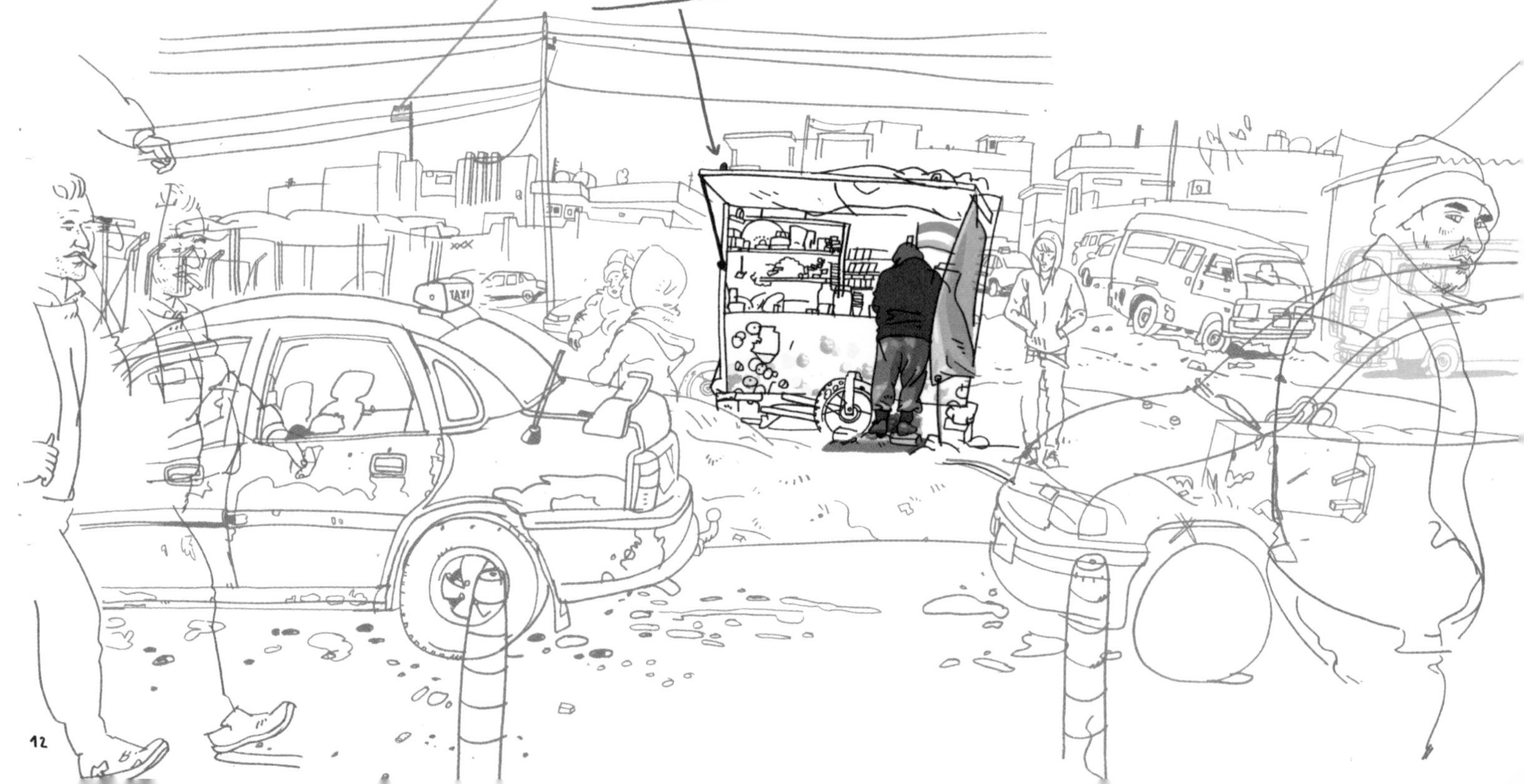
MUHAMED'S TEA CART

MUHAMED 55 YEARS OLD

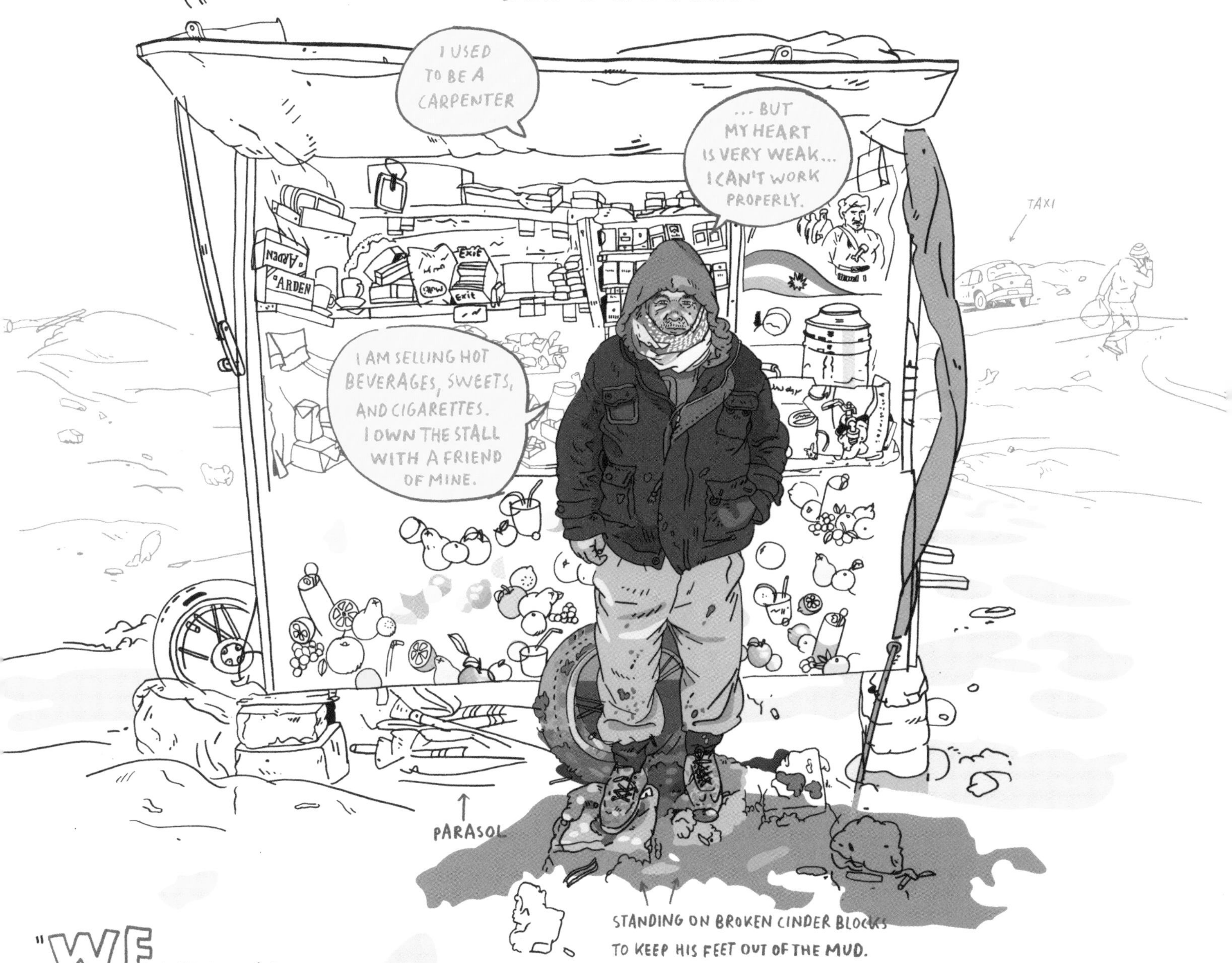
I USED TO BE A CARPENTER
... BUT MY HEART IS VERY WEAK... I CAN'T WORK PROPERLY.
I AM SELLING HOT BEVERAGES, SWEETS, AND CIGARETTES. I OWN THE STALL WITH A FRIEND OF MINE.
TAXI
ARDEN
PARASOL
STANDING ON BROKEN CINDER BLOCKS TO KEEP HIS FEET OUT OF THE MUD.

"WE FLED SYRIA FIFTEEN MONTHS AGO. WE HAD BEEN LIVING IN DAMASCUS FOR MANY YEARS. ONE AFTERNOON WE COULD HEAR A HELICOPTER APPROACHING. IT RANDOMLY STARTED BOMBING HOUSES IN OUR NEIGHBORHOOD. WE RAN AWAY FROM OUR HOUSE JUST IN TIME— IT WAS HIT BY A BOMB AND DESTROYED. IT WAS NOT SAFE TO STAY... AS I'VE GOT SEVEN DAUGHTERS I WAS VERY WORRIED THAT THEY WOULD GET RAPED... WE LEFT DAMASCUS IMMEDIATELY BY BUS WITH NOTHING BUT THE CLOTHES WE'D BEEN WEARING. THE JOURNEY TO QUAMISHLI WAS SCARY AS THERE ARE MANY CHECKPOINTS. THEY ARE MANNED BY EITHER THE SYRIAN ARMY, THE FREE SYRIAN ARMY, OR JIHADIST GROUPS. BUT WE MADE IT AND WERE ABLE TO STAY FOR A WHILE WITH MY FATHER-IN-LAW'S FAMILY. BUT I HAVE A LARGE FAMILY, SO WE COULDN'T STAY WITH THEM FOR LONG. BECAUSE OF THE WAR THERE IS NO WORK IN THE AREA. FOOD, ELECTRICITY, AND FUEL ARE SCARCE AND EXPENSIVE SO WE LEFT FOR IRAQI KURDISTAN. NOW, IN THE CAMP, WE ALL LIVE IN ONE TENT. I AM HAPPY THAT WE ARE ALL TOGETHER BUT I AM NOT HAPPY WITH THE LIVING CONDITIONS HERE... THE RAIN, THE COLD... THERE IS WATER EVERYWHERE. I HAVE A BIG FAMILY TO LOOK AFTER BUT I AM OLD AND I AM SICK..."

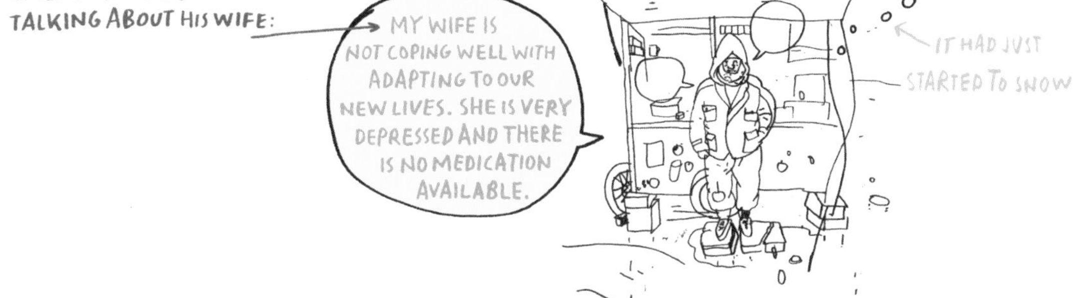
CRIES WHEN HE STARTS TALKING ABOUT HIS WIFE:
MY WIFE IS NOT COPING WELL WITH ADAPTING TO OUR NEW LIVES. SHE IS VERY DEPRESSED AND THERE IS NO MEDICATION AVAILABLE.
IT HAD JUST STARTED TO SNOW

THE PLAYGROUND

BECAUSE THE CAMP SOON BECAME OVERCROWDED, NEW ARRIVALS PITCHED THEIR TENTS IN FRONT OF THE FENCE SECURING THE CAMP'S SOUTHEASTERN BORDER. THIS AREA WAS ORIGINALLY EARMARKED BY THE PLANNERS TO SERVE AS A RECREATIONAL AREA THAT WOULD HAVE INCLUDED A FOOTBALL PITCH AND A PLAYGROUND.

UNHCR
KINDER GUMMI-STIEFEL

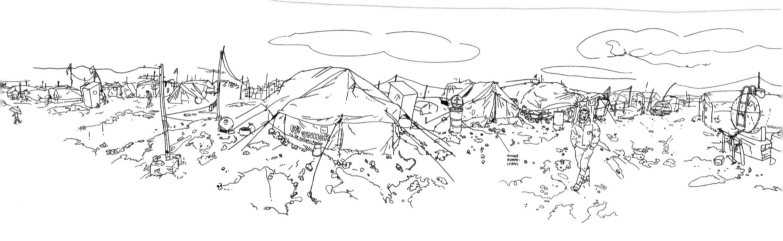

AUTHOR'S NOTE:

Julien, Mazen (our translator) and I had spent the best part of an hour in the family's tent when I noticed some movement underneath the blankets on top of the matress: ⟶
one of Ahmed's teenage sons had been hiding there... Was he embarrassed? I didn't want to ask.

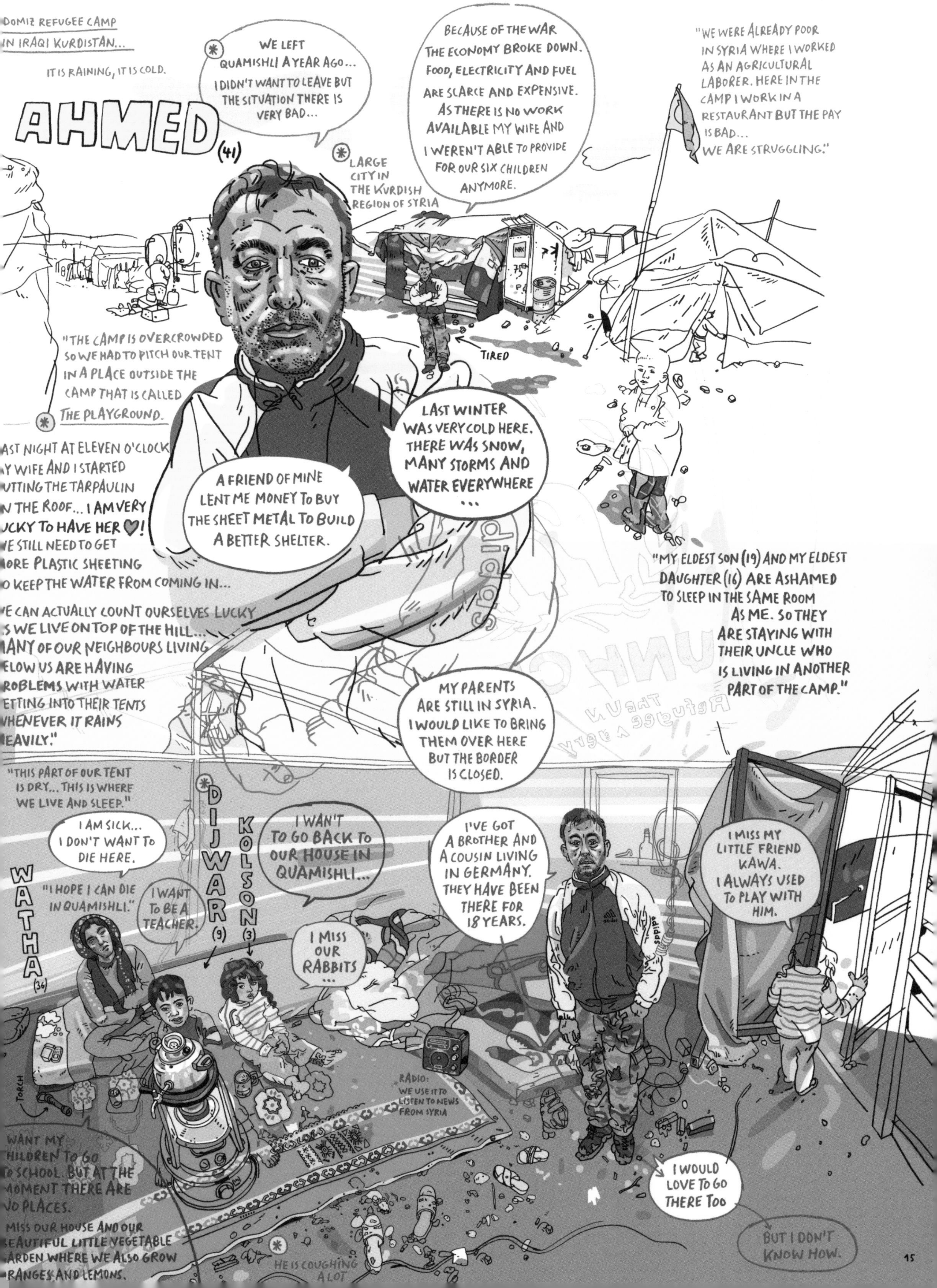
DOMIZ REFUGEE CAMP IN IRAQI KURDISTAN...
IT IS RAINING, IT IS COLD.
AHMED (41)
* WE LEFT QUAMISHLI A YEAR AGO... I DIDN'T WANT TO LEAVE BUT THE SITUATION THERE IS VERY BAD...
* LARGE CITY IN THE KURDISH REGION OF SYRIA
BECAUSE OF THE WAR THE ECONOMY BROKE DOWN. FOOD, ELECTRICITY AND FUEL ARE SCARCE AND EXPENSIVE. AS THERE IS NO WORK AVAILABLE MY WIFE AND I WEREN'T ABLE TO PROVIDE FOR OUR SIX CHILDREN ANYMORE.
"WE WERE ALREADY POOR IN SYRIA WHERE I WORKED AS AN AGRICULTURAL LABORER. HERE IN THE CAMP I WORK IN A RESTAURANT BUT THE PAY IS BAD... WE ARE STRUGGLING."
NRC
TIRED
"THE CAMP IS OVERCROWDED SO WE HAD TO PITCH OUR TENT IN A PLACE OUTSIDE THE CAMP THAT IS CALLED * THE PLAYGROUND.
AST NIGHT AT ELEVEN O'CLOCK Y WIFE AND I STARTED UTTING THE TARPAULIN N THE ROOF... I AM VERY UCKY TO HAVE HER ♥! E STILL NEED TO GET ORE PLASTIC SHEETING O KEEP THE WATER FROM COMING IN...
E CAN ACTUALLY COUNT OURSELVES LUCKY S WE LIVE ON TOP OF THE HILL... ANY OF OUR NEIGHBOURS LIVING ELOW US ARE HAVING ROBLEMS WITH WATER ETTING INTO THEIR TENTS HENEVER IT RAINS EAVILY."
A FRIEND OF MINE LENT ME MONEY TO BUY THE SHEET METAL TO BUILD A BETTER SHELTER.
LAST WINTER WAS VERY COLD HERE. THERE WAS SNOW, MANY STORMS AND WATER EVERYWHERE...
"MY ELDEST SON (19) AND MY ELDEST DAUGHTER (16) ARE ASHAMED TO SLEEP IN THE SAME ROOM AS ME. SO THEY ARE STAYING WITH THEIR UNCLE WHO IS LIVING IN ANOTHER PART OF THE CAMP."
MY PARENTS ARE STILL IN SYRIA. I WOULD LIKE TO BRING THEM OVER HERE BUT THE BORDER IS CLOSED.
"THIS PART OF OUR TENT IS DRY... THIS IS WHERE WE LIVE AND SLEEP."
I AM SICK... I DON'T WANT TO DIE HERE.
"I HOPE I CAN DIE IN QUAMISHLI."
WATHA (36)
I WANT TO BE A TEACHER.
* DIJWAR (9)
KOLSON (3)
I WAN'T TO GO BACK TO OUR HOUSE IN QUAMISHLI...
I MISS OUR RABBITS...
I'VE GOT A BROTHER AND A COUSIN LIVING IN GERMANY. THEY HAVE BEEN THERE FOR 18 YEARS.
I MISS MY LITTLE FRIEND KAWA. I ALWAYS USED TO PLAY WITH HIM.
TORCH
RADIO: WE USE IT TO LISTEN TO NEWS FROM SYRIA
WANT MY HILDREN TO GO O SCHOOL. BUT AT THE MOMENT THERE ARE NO PLACES. MISS OUR HOUSE AND OUR BEAUTIFUL LITTLE VEGETABLE ARDEN WHERE WE ALSO GROW RANGES AND LEMONS.
* HE IS COUGHING A LOT
I WOULD LOVE TO GO THERE TOO
BUT I DON'T KNOW HOW.

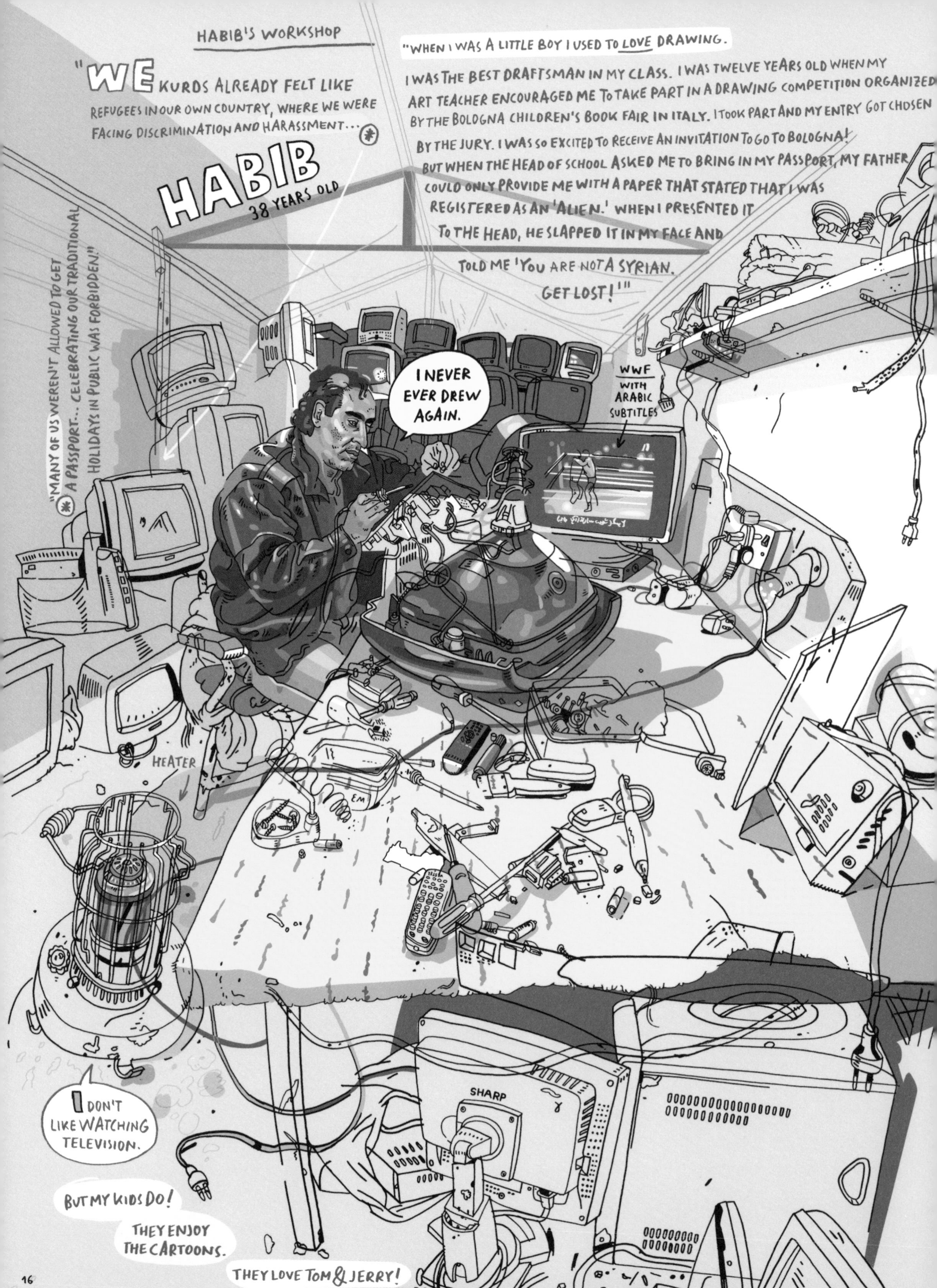
HABIB'S WORKSHOP
"WE KURDS ALREADY FELT LIKE REFUGEES IN OUR OWN COUNTRY, WHERE WE WERE FACING DISCRIMINATION AND HARASSMENT... (*)
HABIB
38 YEARS OLD
"WHEN I WAS A LITTLE BOY I USED TO LOVE DRAWING.
I WAS THE BEST DRAFTSMAN IN MY CLASS. I WAS TWELVE YEARS OLD WHEN MY ART TEACHER ENCOURAGED ME TO TAKE PART IN A DRAWING COMPETITION ORGANIZED BY THE BOLOGNA CHILDREN'S BOOK FAIR IN ITALY. I TOOK PART AND MY ENTRY GOT CHOSEN BY THE JURY. I WAS SO EXCITED TO RECEIVE AN INVITATION TO GO TO BOLOGNA! BUT WHEN THE HEAD OF SCHOOL ASKED ME TO BRING IN MY PASSPORT, MY FATHER COULD ONLY PROVIDE ME WITH A PAPER THAT STATED THAT I WAS REGISTERED AS AN 'ALIEN.' WHEN I PRESENTED IT TO THE HEAD, HE SLAPPED IT IN MY FACE AND TOLD ME 'YOU ARE NOT A SYRIAN. GET LOST!'"
(*) "MANY OF US WEREN'T ALLOWED TO GET A PASSPORT... CELEBRATING OUR TRADITIONAL HOLIDAYS IN PUBLIC WAS FORBIDDEN!"
I NEVER EVER DREW AGAIN.
WWF WITH ARABIC SUBTITLES
HEATER
SHARP
I DON'T LIKE WATCHING TELEVISION.
BUT MY KIDS DO!
THEY ENJOY THE CARTOONS.
THEY LOVE TOM & JERRY!

"WE'VE BEEN LIVING HERE IN DOMIZ FOR ABOUT ONE AND A HALF YEARS. LAST YEAR MY BROTHER-IN-LAW AND I BOUGHT SOME BUILDING MATERIALS AND STARTED TO BUILD US A SMALL LITTLE HOUSE AND THIS WORKSHOP. IT IS NOT FINISHED YET BUT IT SHOULD GET US THROUGH THE WINTER.

"I'VE ALWAYS BEEN FASCINATED BY ELECTRICAL APPLIANCES. WHENEVER MY PARENTS BOUGHT A NEW RECORD PLAYER OR RADIO IT DIDN'T TAKE LONG UNTIL I GOT MY HANDS ON IT AND EVENTUALLY BROKE IT. WHEN I WAS ABOUT TEN YEARS OLD I STARTED TO VISIT THE WORKSHOP RUN BY A FRIEND OF MY FATHER. HE TAUGHT ME HOW TO REPAIR ELECTRICAL APPLIANCES. THIS BECAME MY HOBBY AND LATER MY JOB.

"I WANT TO TRAVEL TO EUROPE. AS I DON'T HAVE A PASSPORT I CAN'T DO IT LEGALLY. FIFTEEN YEARS AGO I PAID A TRAFFICKER 5,000 US DOLLARS TO TAKE ME TO CYPRUS AND FROM THERE ON TO ITALY... IT TURNED OUT HE WAS A CHEAT AND RAN AWAY WITH THE MONEY. I TRIED IT AGAIN A COUPLE MORE TIMES BUT NO LUCK! AFTERWARDS I GOT MARRIED AND HAD CHILDREN."

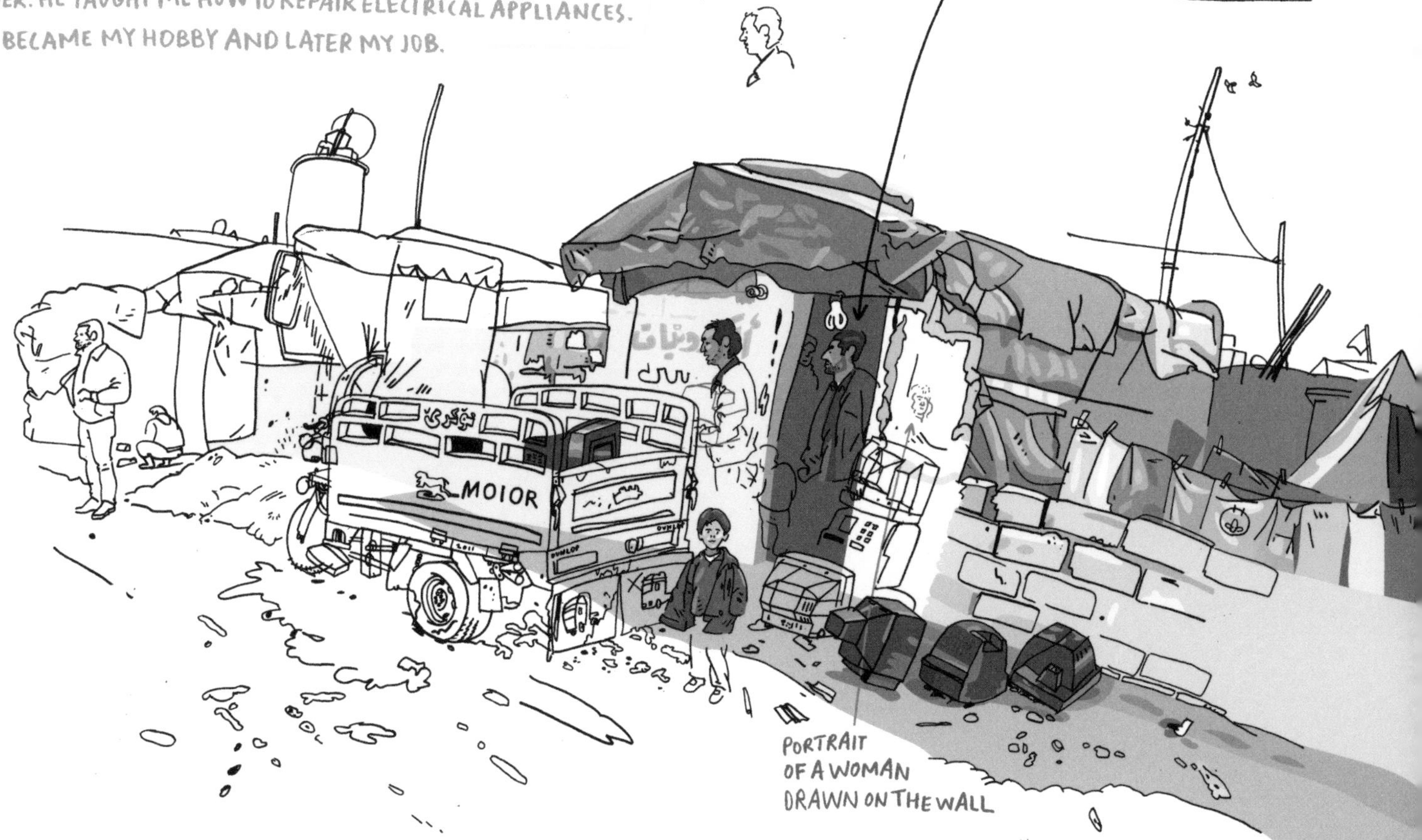

A CUSTOMER AND HIS SON PICKING UP A REPAIRED TV SET
MOTOR
PORTRAIT OF A WOMAN DRAWN ON THE WALL

"ONE OF MY OTHER PASSIONS IS MUSIC. IN DAMASCUS I ALSO USED TO WORK AS A MUSICIAN. MY SIBLINGS AND I USED TO EARN GOOD MONEY PLAYING AT WEDDINGS AND OTHER PARTIES. I ESPECIALLY ENJOYED PLAYING THE TAMBOUR.(*) I ALSO USED TO PERFORM IN A CASINO. THERE, THOUGH WE HAD TO PLAY ARABIC MUSIC AS OUR KURDISH MUSIC WAS NOT WELCOMED.

"WHEN THE WAR STARTED I DIDN'T SEE ANY FUTURE FOR MY FAMILY IN OUR COUNTRY. AGAIN, WE DECIDED TO GO TO EUROPE. I PAID A TRAFFICKER TO TAKE US TO TURKEY AND FROM THERE TO GREECE... IT TURNED OUT, AGAIN, THAT THE GUY WAS A FRAUD. WITH NO SAVINGS LEFT, WE HAD TO SELL MY WIFE'S JEWELLERY IN ORDER TO FLEE TO (IRAQI →) KURDISTAN.

"WE ARE FORTUNATE IN BEING WELCOMED BY OUR BROTHERS IN KURDISTAN BUT I DON'T SEE ANY FUTURE FOR US HERE EITHER. I DON'T PLAY MUSIC ANYMORE AS I DON'T FEEL HAPPY. INSTEAD I WORK HERE IN MY SHOP. THERE IS A LOT OF DEMAND AND MY WORK IS WELL RESPECTED. I USUALLY WORK UNTIL MIDNIGHT... I WANT TO SAVE MONEY... BUT I ALSO REPAIR APPLIANCES FOR FREE IF THE CUSTOMER HAS GOT NO MONEY.

"A COUSIN OF MINE LIVES IN BULGARIA WHERE HE IS DOING QUITE WELL. HE TOLD ME IT IS RELATIVELY EASY AND SAFE TO GET THERE. MAYBE NEXT YEAR OR THE YEAR AFTER WE WILL GO TO EUROPE, INSHALLAH."

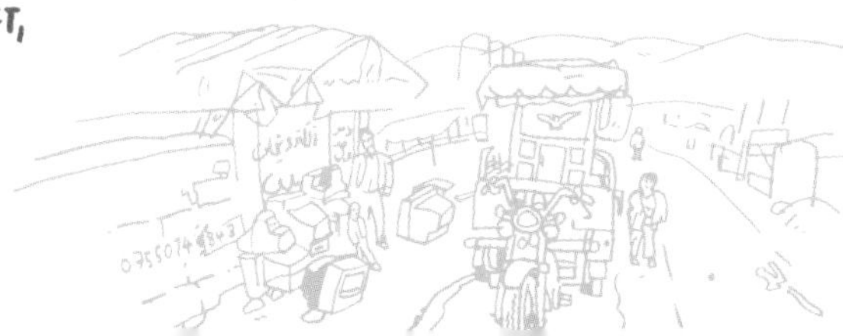

(*) KURDISH TRADITIONAL INSTRUMENT... → A LONG NECKED LUTE.

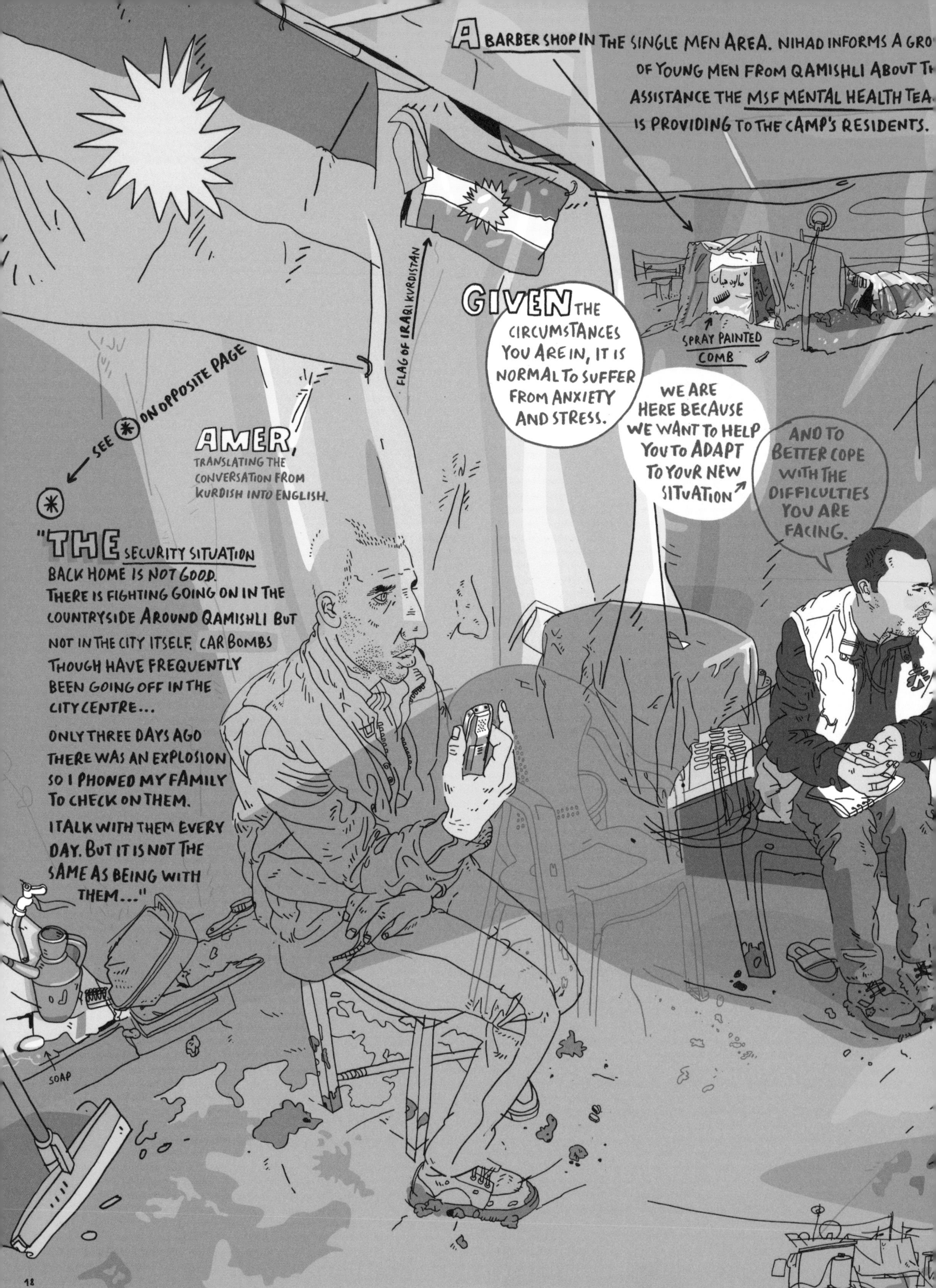

A BARBER SHOP IN THE SINGLE MEN AREA. NIHAD INFORMS A GRO OF YOUNG MEN FROM QAMISHLI ABOUT TH ASSISTANCE THE MSF MENTAL HEALTH TEA IS PROVIDING TO THE CAMP'S RESIDENTS.
FLAG OF IRAQI KURDISTAN
SPRAY PAINTED COMB
GIVEN THE CIRCUMSTANCES YOU ARE IN, IT IS NORMAL TO SUFFER FROM ANXIETY AND STRESS.
WE ARE HERE BECAUSE WE WANT TO HELP YOU TO ADAPT TO YOUR NEW SITUATION
AND TO BETTER COPE WITH THE DIFFICULTIES YOU ARE FACING.
SEE * ON OPPOSITE PAGE
AMER, TRANSLATING THE CONVERSATION FROM KURDISH INTO ENGLISH.
* "THE SECURITY SITUATION BACK HOME IS NOT GOOD. THERE IS FIGHTING GOING ON IN THE COUNTRYSIDE AROUND QAMISHLI BUT NOT IN THE CITY ITSELF. CAR BOMBS THOUGH HAVE FREQUENTLY BEEN GOING OFF IN THE CITY CENTRE...
ONLY THREE DAYS AGO THERE WAS AN EXPLOSION SO I PHONED MY FAMILY TO CHECK ON THEM.
I TALK WITH THEM EVERY DAY. BUT IT IS NOT THE SAME AS BEING WITH THEM..."
SOAP

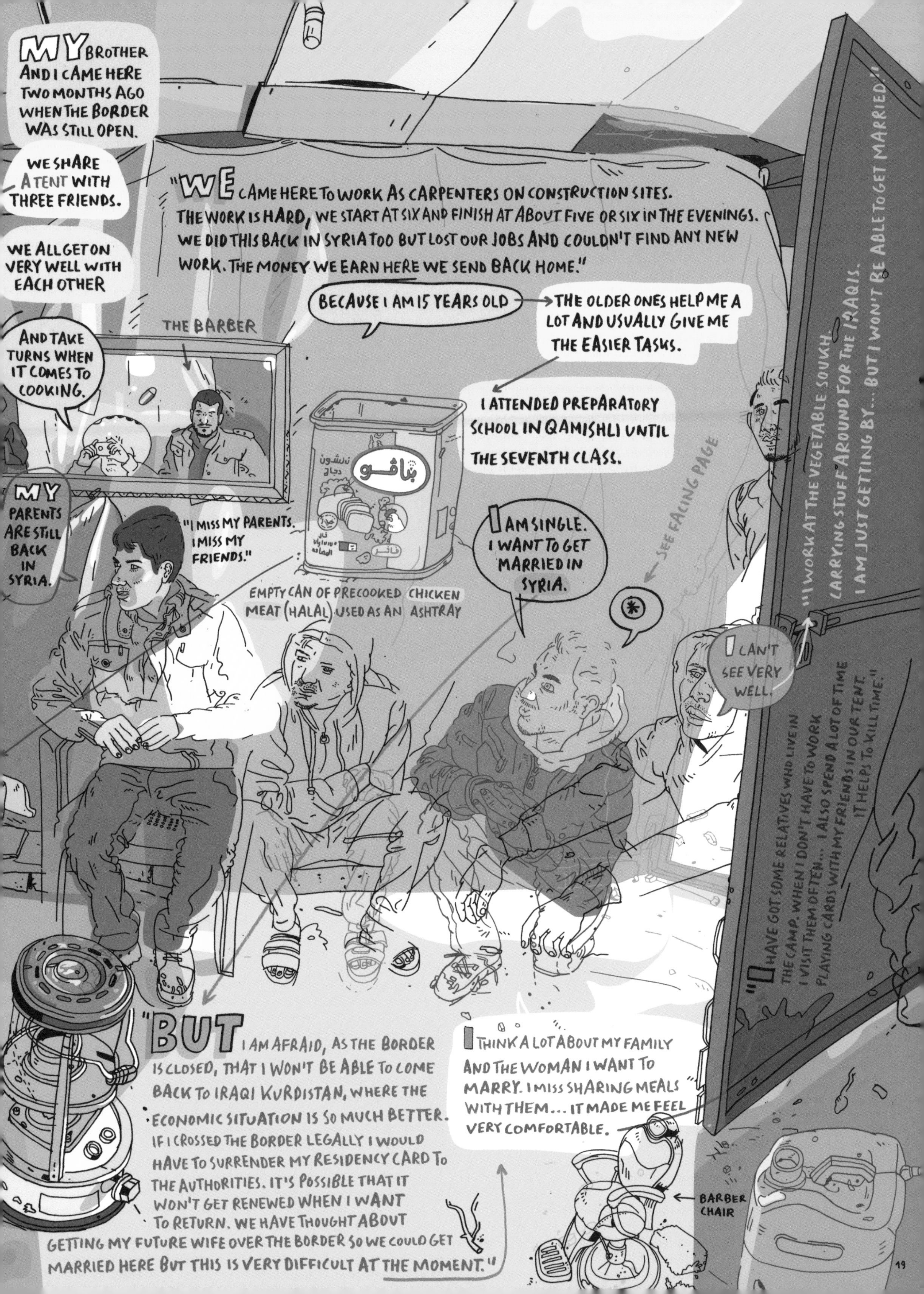

MY BROTHER AND I CAME HERE TWO MONTHS AGO WHEN THE BORDER WAS STILL OPEN.
WE SHARE A TENT WITH THREE FRIENDS.
WE ALL GET ON VERY WELL WITH EACH OTHER
AND TAKE TURNS WHEN IT COMES TO COOKING.
"WE CAME HERE TO WORK AS CARPENTERS ON CONSTRUCTION SITES. THE WORK IS HARD, WE START AT SIX AND FINISH AT ABOUT FIVE OR SIX IN THE EVENINGS. WE DID THIS BACK IN SYRIA TOO BUT LOST OUR JOBS AND COULDN'T FIND ANY NEW WORK. THE MONEY WE EARN HERE WE SEND BACK HOME."
BECAUSE I AM 15 YEARS OLD
THE OLDER ONES HELP ME A LOT AND USUALLY GIVE ME THE EASIER TASKS.
I ATTENDED PREPARATORY SCHOOL IN QAMISHLI UNTIL THE SEVENTH CLASS.
THE BARBER
MY PARENTS ARE STILL BACK IN SYRIA.
"I MISS MY PARENTS. I MISS MY FRIENDS."
EMPTY CAN OF PRECOOKED CHICKEN MEAT (HALAL) USED AS AN ASHTRAY
I AM SINGLE. I WANT TO GET MARRIED IN SYRIA.
SEE FACING PAGE
*
I CAN'T SEE VERY WELL.
"I WORK AT THE VEGETABLE SOUKH. CARRYING STUFF AROUND FOR THE IRAQIS. I AM JUST GETTING BY... BUT I WON'T BE ABLE TO GET MARRIED."
"I HAVE GOT SOME RELATIVES WHO LIVE IN THE CAMP. WHEN I DON'T HAVE TO WORK I VISIT THEM OFTEN... I ALSO SPEND A LOT OF TIME PLAYING CARDS WITH MY FRIENDS IN OUR TENT. IT HELPS TO KILL TIME."
"BUT I AM AFRAID, AS THE BORDER IS CLOSED, THAT I WON'T BE ABLE TO COME BACK TO IRAQI KURDISTAN, WHERE THE ECONOMIC SITUATION IS SO MUCH BETTER. IF I CROSSED THE BORDER LEGALLY I WOULD HAVE TO SURRENDER MY RESIDENCY CARD TO THE AUTHORITIES. IT'S POSSIBLE THAT IT WON'T GET RENEWED WHEN I WANT TO RETURN. WE HAVE THOUGHT ABOUT GETTING MY FUTURE WIFE OVER THE BORDER SO WE COULD GET MARRIED HERE BUT THIS IS VERY DIFFICULT AT THE MOMENT."
I THINK A LOT ABOUT MY FAMILY AND THE WOMAN I WANT TO MARRY. I MISS SHARING MEALS WITH THEM... IT MADE ME FEEL VERY COMFORTABLE.
BARBER CHAIR

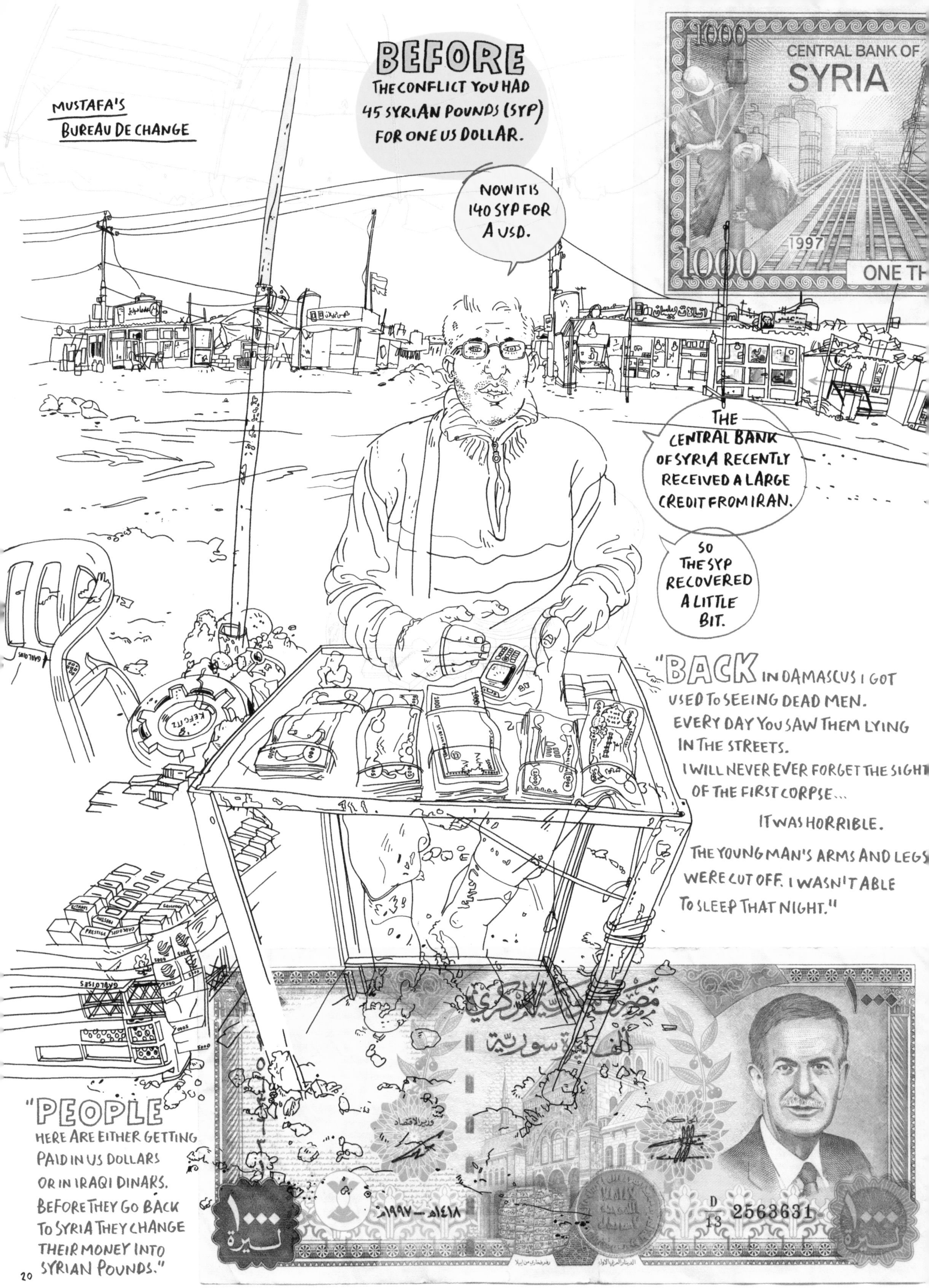
MUSTAFA'S BUREAU DE CHANGE
BEFORE THE CONFLICT YOU HAD 45 SYRIAN POUNDS (SYP) FOR ONE US DOLLAR.
NOW IT IS 140 SYP FOR A USD.
THE CENTRAL BANK OF SYRIA RECENTLY RECEIVED A LARGE CREDIT FROM IRAN.
SO THE SYP RECOVERED A LITTLE BIT.
"BACK IN DAMASCUS I GOT USED TO SEEING DEAD MEN. EVERY DAY YOU SAW THEM LYING IN THE STREETS. I WILL NEVER EVER FORGET THE SIGHT OF THE FIRST CORPSE... IT WAS HORRIBLE. THE YOUNG MAN'S ARMS AND LEGS WERE CUT OFF. I WASN'T ABLE TO SLEEP THAT NIGHT."
"PEOPLE HERE ARE EITHER GETTING PAID IN US DOLLARS OR IN IRAQI DINARS. BEFORE THEY GO BACK TO SYRIA THEY CHANGE THEIR MONEY INTO SYRIAN POUNDS."
CENTRAL BANK OF
SYRIA
1000
1997
ONE TH
2563631

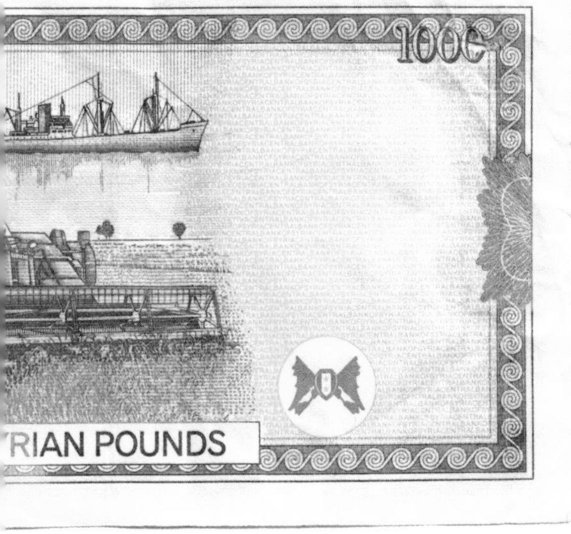
1000
RIAN POUNDS

AUTHOR'S NOTE:

When we arrived ISSA invited us to smoke his Shisha pipe with him. Not like any Shisha I had encountered before, but one that was fondly and lovingly decorated with fresh fruit: oranges, plums, apples and pomegranates. Like something straight out of the Arabian Nights.

A'S BARBER SHOP

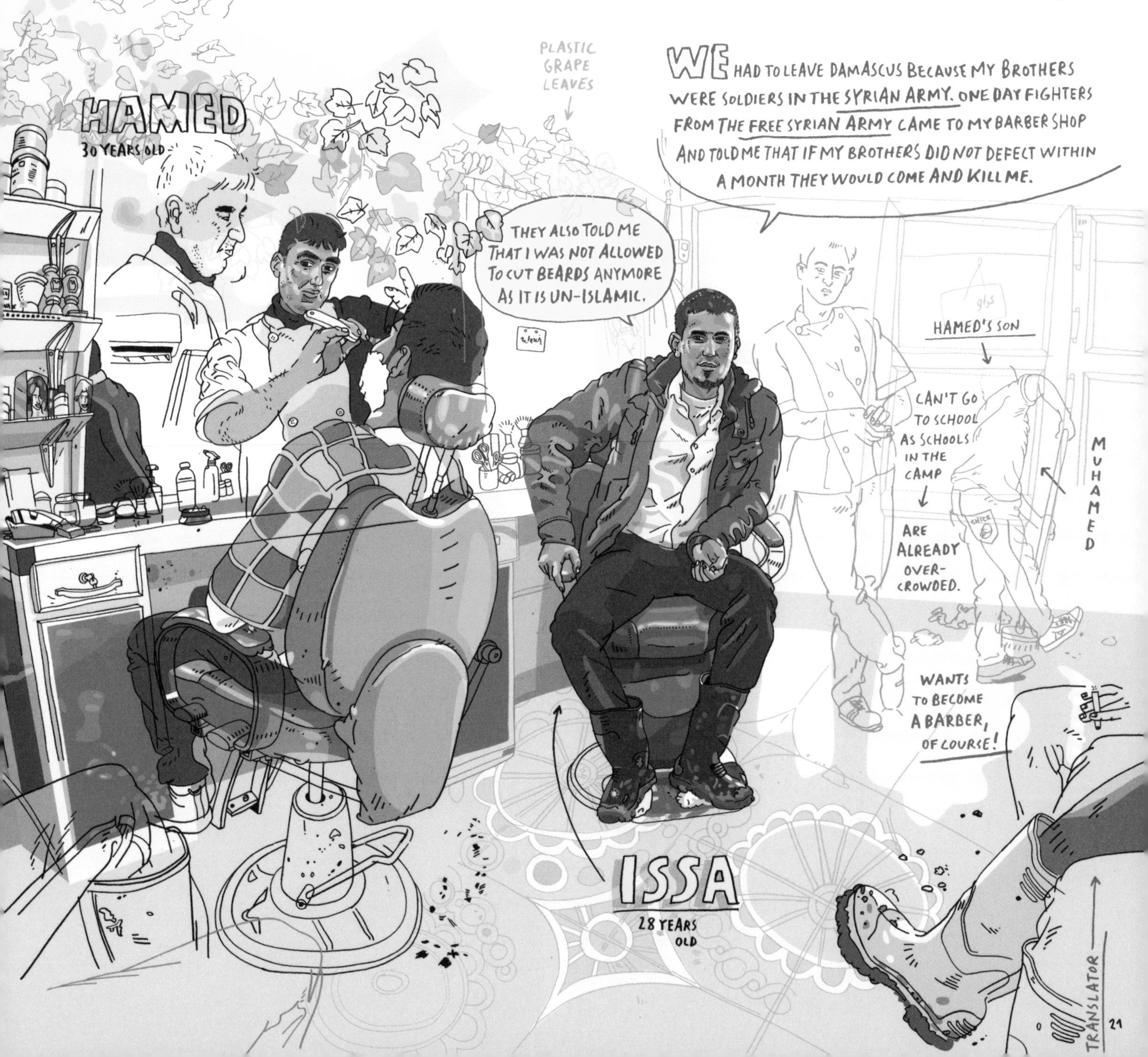
HAMED
30 YEARS OLD
PLASTIC GRAPE LEAVES
WE HAD TO LEAVE DAMASCUS BECAUSE MY BROTHERS WERE SOLDIERS IN THE SYRIAN ARMY. ONE DAY FIGHTERS FROM THE FREE SYRIAN ARMY CAME TO MY BARBER SHOP AND TOLD ME THAT IF MY BROTHERS DID NOT DEFECT WITHIN A MONTH THEY WOULD COME AND KILL ME.
THEY ALSO TOLD ME THAT I WAS NOT ALLOWED TO CUT BEARDS ANYMORE AS IT IS UN-ISLAMIC.
HAMED'S SON
CAN'T GO TO SCHOOL AS SCHOOLS IN THE CAMP ARE ALREADY OVER-CROWDED.
MUHAMED
WANTS TO BECOME A BARBER, OF COURSE!
ISSA
28 YEARS OLD
TRANSLATOR

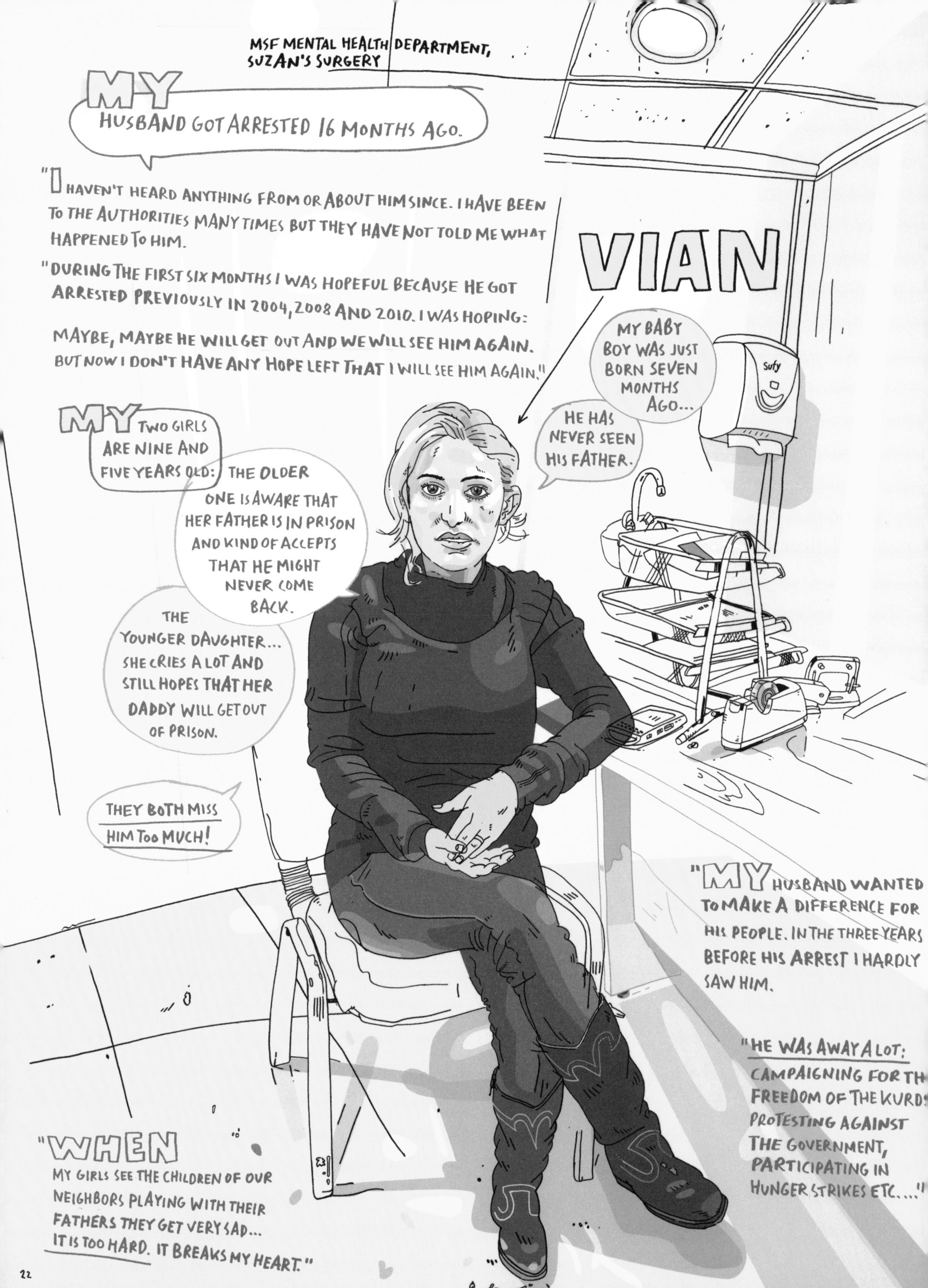
MSF MENTAL HEALTH DEPARTMENT, SUZAN'S SURGERY
MY HUSBAND GOT ARRESTED 16 MONTHS AGO.
"I HAVEN'T HEARD ANYTHING FROM OR ABOUT HIM SINCE. I HAVE BEEN TO THE AUTHORITIES MANY TIMES BUT THEY HAVE NOT TOLD ME WHAT HAPPENED TO HIM.
"DURING THE FIRST SIX MONTHS I WAS HOPEFUL BECAUSE HE GOT ARRESTED PREVIOUSLY IN 2004, 2008 AND 2010. I WAS HOPING:
MAYBE, MAYBE HE WILL GET OUT AND WE WILL SEE HIM AGAIN. BUT NOW I DON'T HAVE ANY HOPE LEFT THAT I WILL SEE HIM AGAIN."
VIAN
MY BABY BOY WAS JUST BORN SEVEN MONTHS AGO...
HE HAS NEVER SEEN HIS FATHER.
Sufy
MY TWO GIRLS ARE NINE AND FIVE YEARS OLD:
THE OLDER ONE IS AWARE THAT HER FATHER IS IN PRISON AND KIND OF ACCEPTS THAT HE MIGHT NEVER COME BACK.
THE YOUNGER DAUGHTER... SHE CRIES A LOT AND STILL HOPES THAT HER DADDY WILL GET OUT OF PRISON.
THEY BOTH MISS HIM TOO MUCH!
"MY HUSBAND WANTED TO MAKE A DIFFERENCE FOR HIS PEOPLE. IN THE THREE YEARS BEFORE HIS ARREST I HARDLY SAW HIM.
"HE WAS AWAY A LOT: CAMPAIGNING FOR THE FREEDOM OF THE KURDS PROTESTING AGAINST THE GOVERNMENT, PARTICIPATING IN HUNGER STRIKES ETC...."
"WHEN MY GIRLS SEE THE CHILDREN OF OUR NEIGHBORS PLAYING WITH THEIR FATHERS THEY GET VERY SAD... IT IS TOO HARD. IT BREAKS MY HEART."

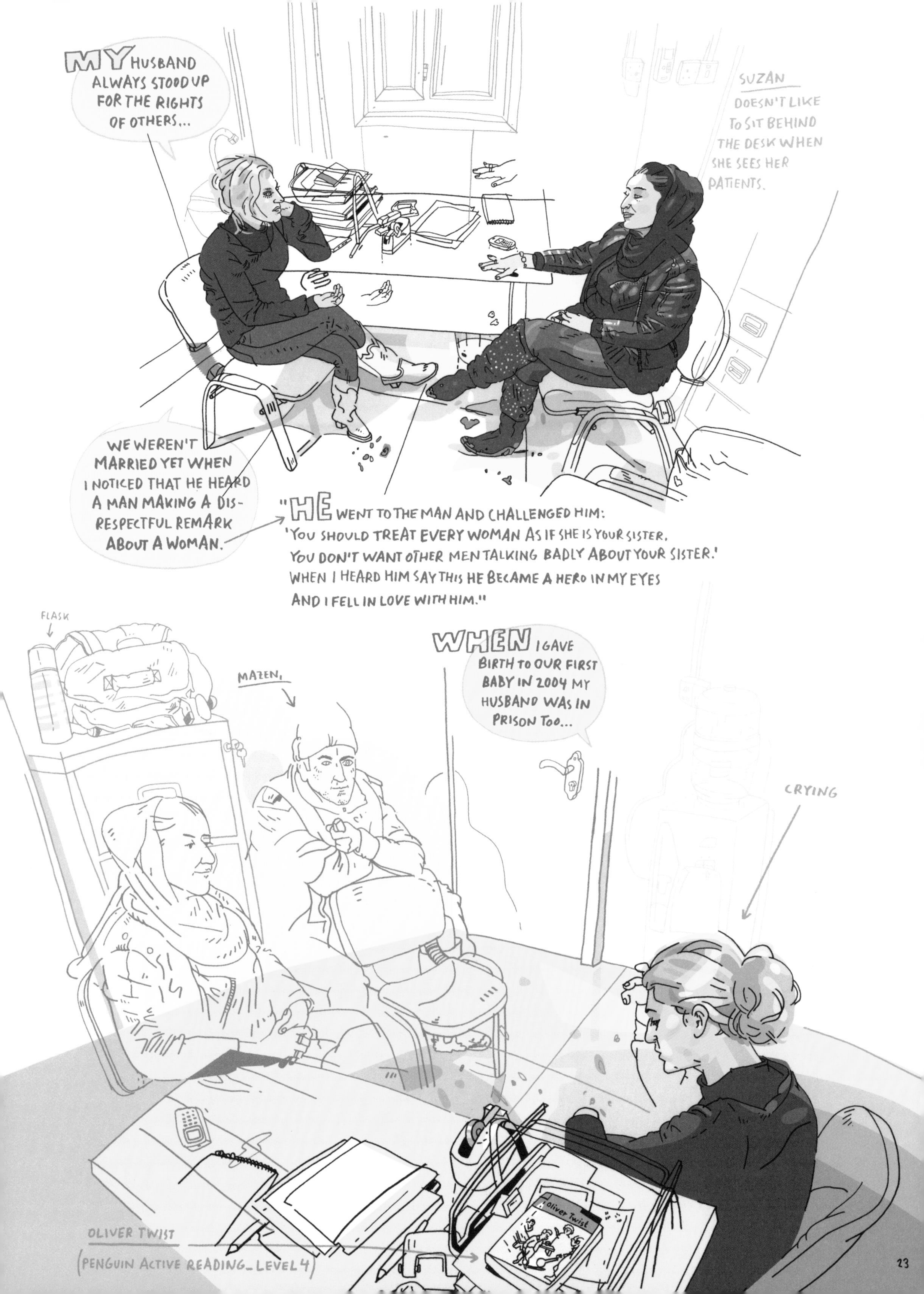
MY HUSBAND ALWAYS STOOD UP FOR THE RIGHTS OF OTHERS...
SUZAN DOESN'T LIKE TO SIT BEHIND THE DESK WHEN SHE SEES HER PATIENTS.
WE WEREN'T MARRIED YET WHEN I NOTICED THAT HE HEARD A MAN MAKING A DISRESPECTFUL REMARK ABOUT A WOMAN.
"HE WENT TO THE MAN AND CHALLENGED HIM: 'YOU SHOULD TREAT EVERY WOMAN AS IF SHE IS YOUR SISTER. YOU DON'T WANT OTHER MEN TALKING BADLY ABOUT YOUR SISTER.' WHEN I HEARD HIM SAY THIS HE BECAME A HERO IN MY EYES AND I FELL IN LOVE WITH HIM."
FLASK
MAZEN,
WHEN I GAVE BIRTH TO OUR FIRST BABY IN 2004 MY HUSBAND WAS IN PRISON TOO...
CRYING
Oliver Twist
OLIVER TWIST
(PENGUIN ACTIVE READING_LEVEL 4)

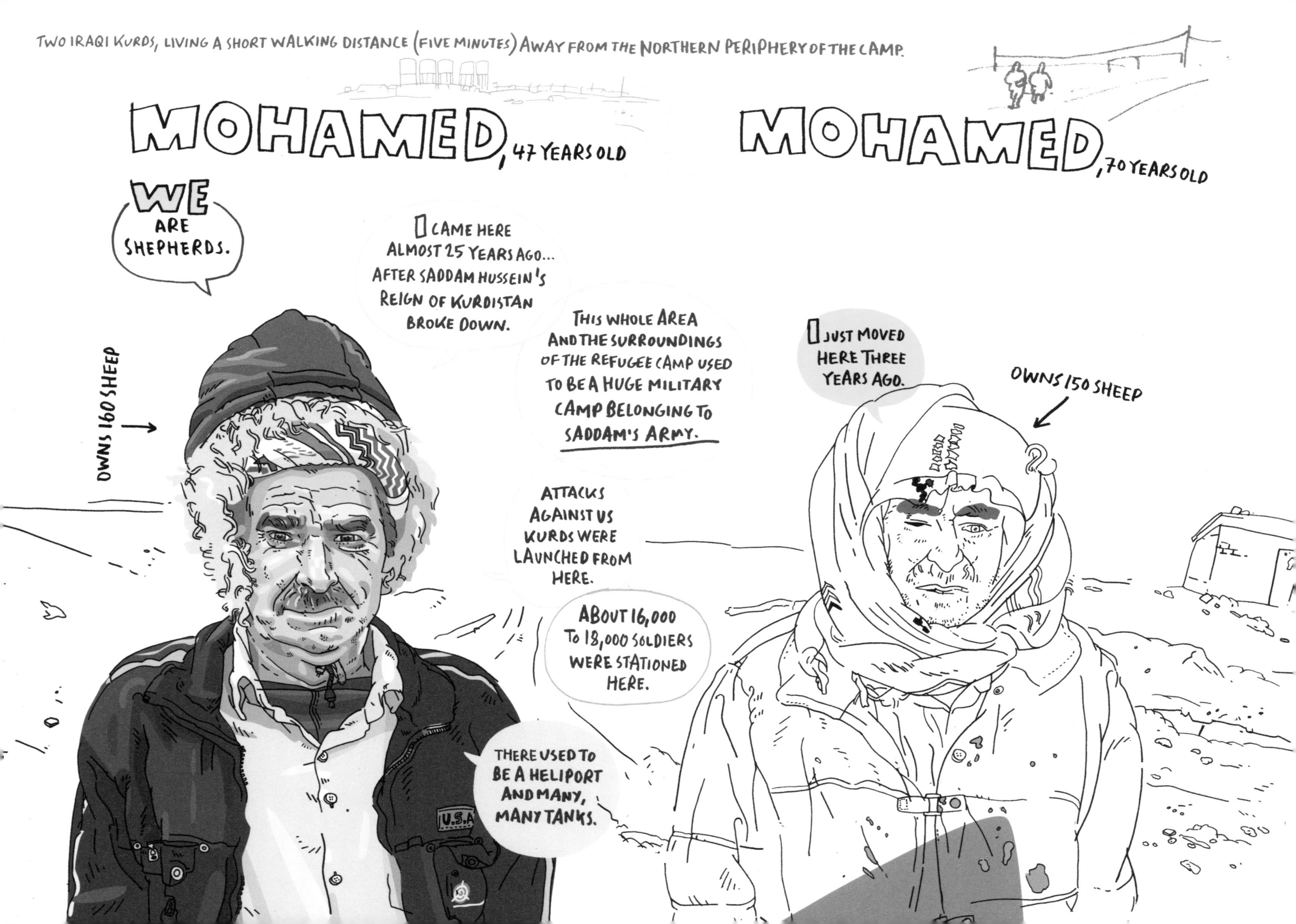
TWO IRAQI KURDS, LIVING A SHORT WALKING DISTANCE (FIVE MINUTES) AWAY FROM THE NORTHERN PERIPHERY OF THE CAMP.
MOHAMED, 47 YEARS OLD
MOHAMED, 70 YEARS OLD
WE ARE SHEPHERDS.
OWNS 160 SHEEP
I CAME HERE ALMOST 25 YEARS AGO... AFTER SADDAM HUSSEIN'S REIGN OF KURDISTAN BROKE DOWN.
THIS WHOLE AREA AND THE SURROUNDINGS OF THE REFUGEE CAMP USED TO BE A HUGE MILITARY CAMP BELONGING TO SADDAM'S ARMY.
ATTACKS AGAINST US KURDS WERE LAUNCHED FROM HERE.
ABOUT 16,000 TO 18,000 SOLDIERS WERE STATIONED HERE.
THERE USED TO BE A HELIPORT AND MANY, MANY TANKS.
I JUST MOVED HERE THREE YEARS AGO.
OWNS 150 SHEEP
U.S.A

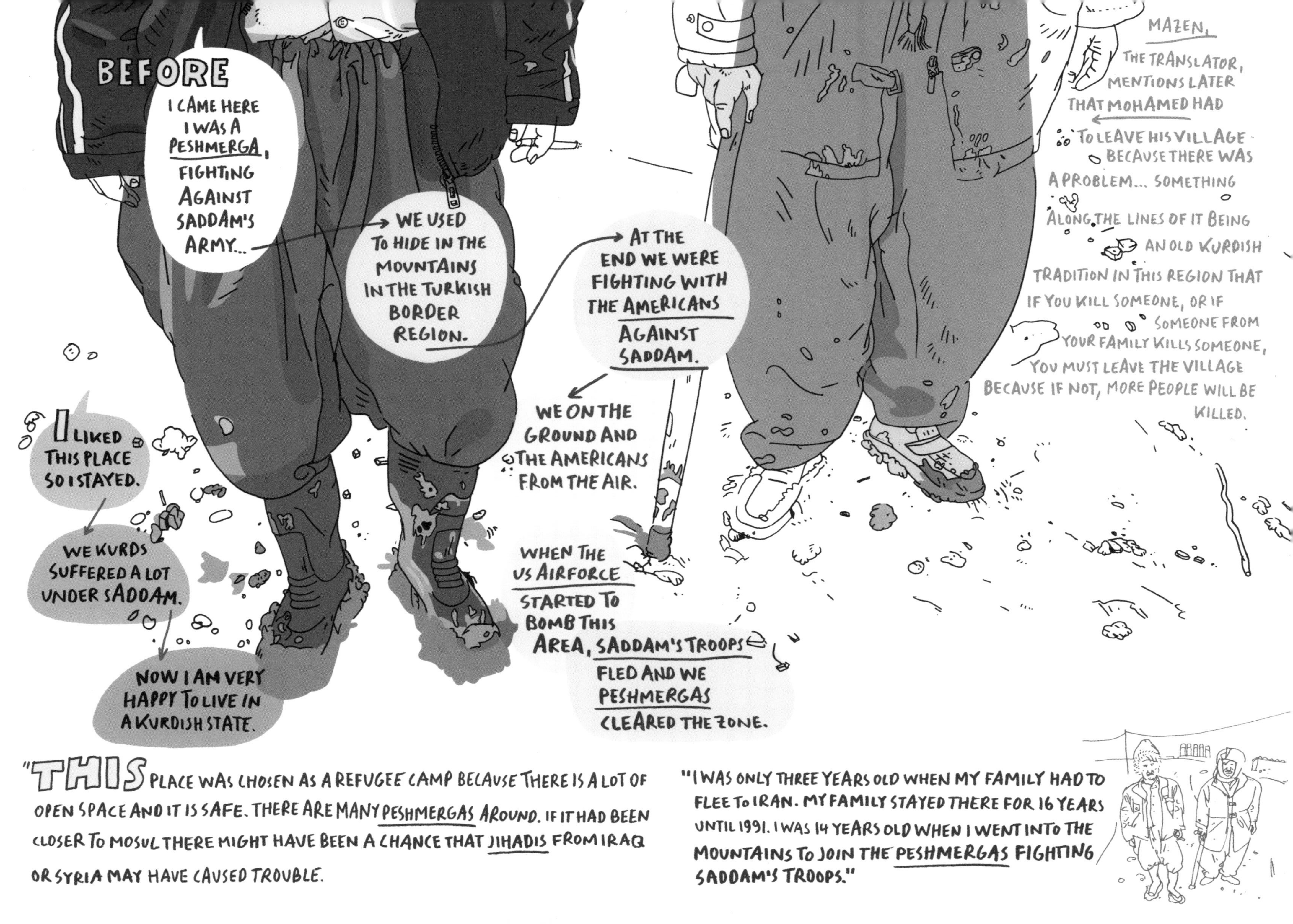
BEFORE I CAME HERE I WAS A PESHMERGA, FIGHTING AGAINST SADDAM'S ARMY...
WE USED TO HIDE IN THE MOUNTAINS IN THE TURKISH BORDER REGION.
AT THE END WE WERE FIGHTING WITH THE AMERICANS AGAINST SADDAM.
WE ON THE GROUND AND THE AMERICANS FROM THE AIR.
WHEN THE US AIRFORCE STARTED TO BOMB THIS AREA, SADDAM'S TROOPS FLED AND WE PESHMERGAS CLEARED THE ZONE.
I LIKED THIS PLACE SO I STAYED.
WE KURDS SUFFERED A LOT UNDER SADDAM.
NOW I AM VERY HAPPY TO LIVE IN A KURDISH STATE.
MAZEN, THE TRANSLATOR, MENTIONS LATER THAT MOHAMED HAD TO LEAVE HIS VILLAGE BECAUSE THERE WAS A PROBLEM... SOMETHING ALONG THE LINES OF IT BEING AN OLD KURDISH TRADITION IN THIS REGION THAT IF YOU KILL SOMEONE, OR IF SOMEONE FROM YOUR FAMILY KILLS SOMEONE, YOU MUST LEAVE THE VILLAGE BECAUSE IF NOT, MORE PEOPLE WILL BE KILLED.
"THIS PLACE WAS CHOSEN AS A REFUGEE CAMP BECAUSE THERE IS A LOT OF OPEN SPACE AND IT IS SAFE. THERE ARE MANY PESHMERGAS AROUND. IF IT HAD BEEN CLOSER TO MOSUL THERE MIGHT HAVE BEEN A CHANCE THAT JIHADIS FROM IRAQ OR SYRIA MAY HAVE CAUSED TROUBLE.
"I WAS ONLY THREE YEARS OLD WHEN MY FAMILY HAD TO FLEE TO IRAN. MY FAMILY STAYED THERE FOR 16 YEARS UNTIL 1991. I WAS 14 YEARS OLD WHEN I WENT INTO THE MOUNTAINS TO JOIN THE PESHMERGAS FIGHTING SADDAM'S TROOPS."

DJWAN'S SOUND SYSTEM RENTAL

TWO ARMCHAIRS COVERED WITH A BLANKET
THE BUSINESS IS GOING OK ...
GIRL DANCING (THE MUSIC HASN'T STARTED YET)

"I RENT OUT THE SYSTEM ABOUT TWICE A WEEK, WHEN THERE IS A WEDDING, A BIRTHDAY PARTY OR WHEN A BABY IS BORN.

"WE GET BETWEEN 75,000 IQD* AND 100,000 IQD (51 GBP) FOR EACH RENTAL.

*IRAQI DINAR

"I DON'T OWN THE BUSINESS... SETTING IT UP THOUGH WAS MY IDEA. AS I DIDN'T HAVE ANY MONEY A FRIEND OF MINE BOUGHT THE EQUIPMENT ABOUT A MONTH AGO FOR ABOUT 3,500 US DOLLARS AND THEN EMPLOYED ME TO RENT IT OUT AND TO OPERATE IT.

"I HAVE ALWAYS BEEN INTERESTED IN MUSIC. I COME FROM AN ARTISTIC FAMILY. HMMM... OK, MY FATHER AND MOTHER LIKE ART... OR AT LEAST THEY DON'T DISLIKE IT. MY BROTHERS AND I, OUR WHOLE FAMILY, WE USED TO SING A LOT WHEN WE WERE YOUNGER. NONE OF US WAS ANY GOOD AT SINGING BUT WE REALLY LOVED DOING IT!

"THE TRADITION WANTS IT THAT THE BRIDE SITS ON THE LEFT HAND SIDE AND THE GROOM ON THE RIGHT HAND SIDE."

"I DO LIKE ALL KINDS OF MUSIC BUT MY FAVOURITE SINGER IS MUHAMMAD SHEKHO, A VERY POPULAR SINGER FROM QUAMISHLI WHERE I GREW UP."

AUTHOR'S NOTE:

One late afternoon at the camp's north-western perimeter, we met a young man setting up a sound system for a wedding celebration. We were only able to have a brief chat with him as we had to leave soon (MSF employees are required to leave the camp before night fall).

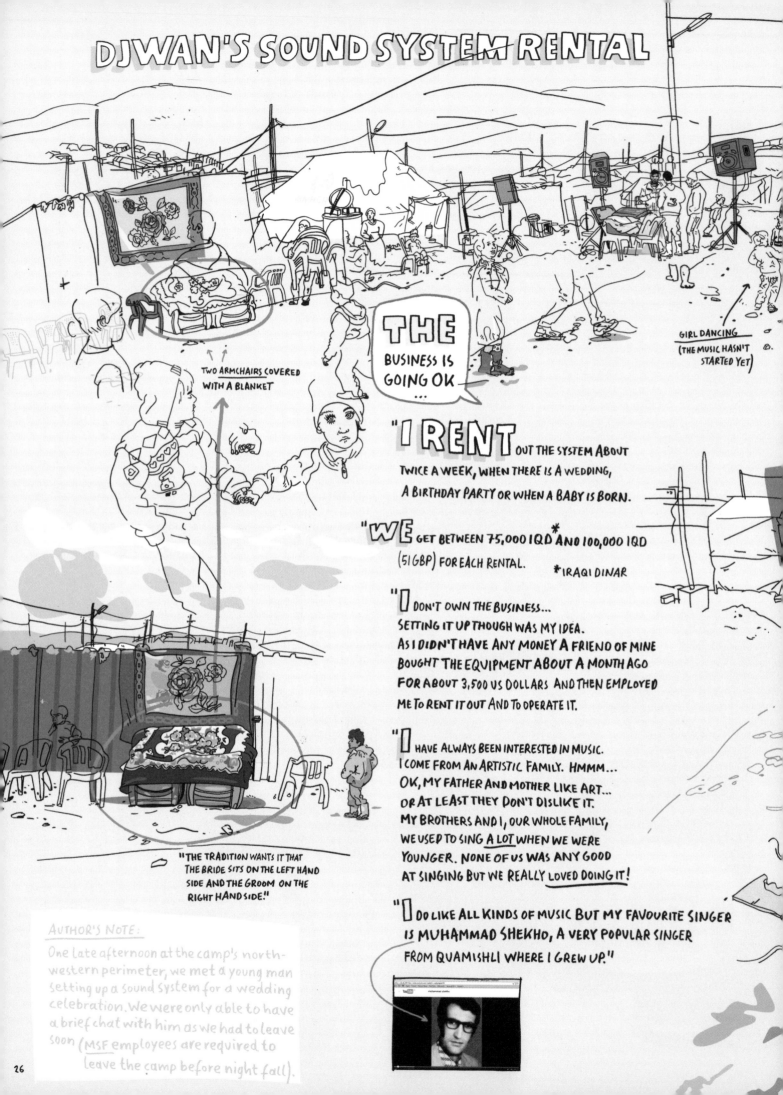

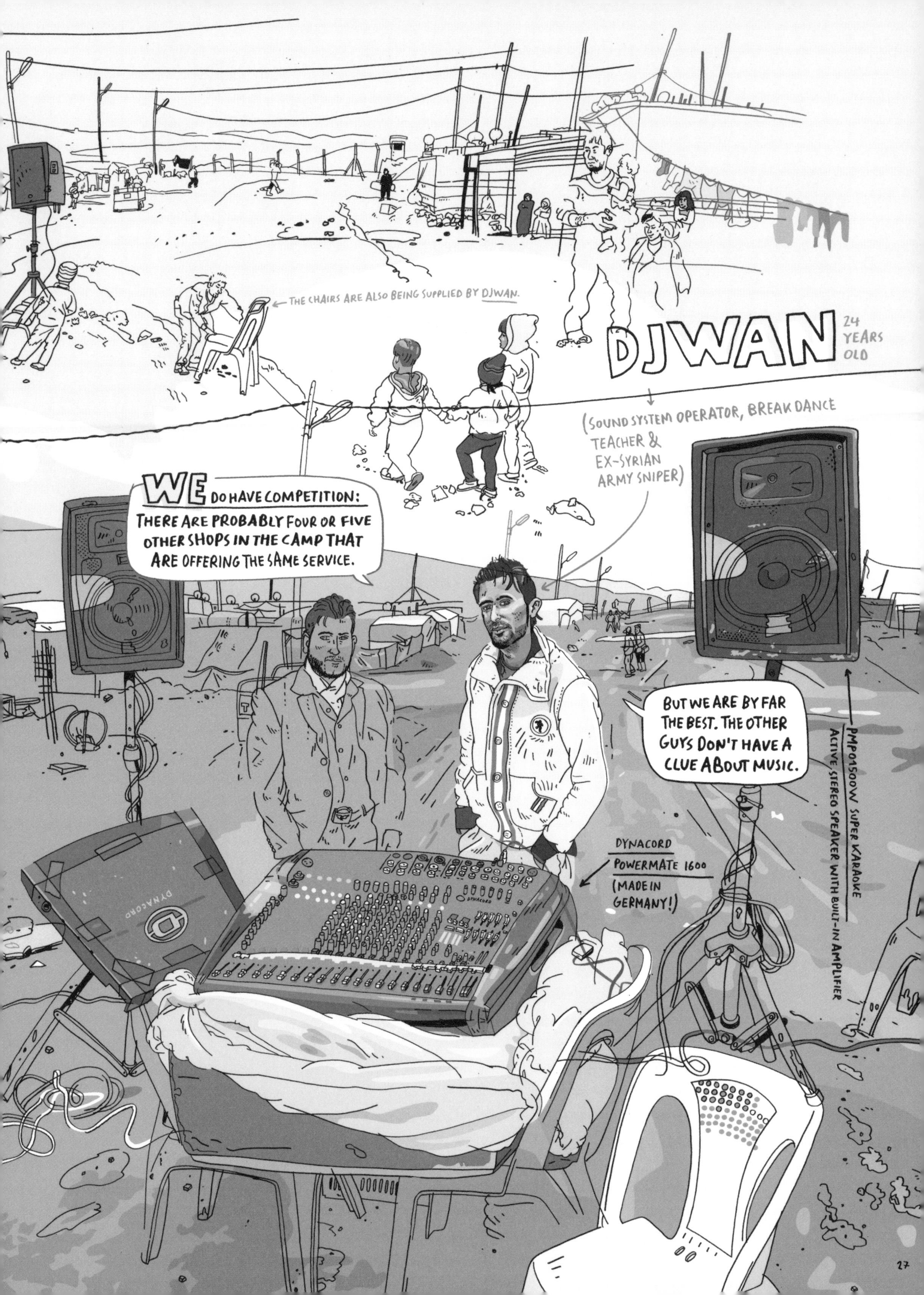

THE CHAIRS ARE ALSO BEING SUPPLIED BY DJWAN.
DJWAN 24 YEARS OLD
(SOUND SYSTEM OPERATOR, BREAK DANCE TEACHER & EX-SYRIAN ARMY SNIPER)
WE DO HAVE COMPETITION: THERE ARE PROBABLY FOUR OR FIVE OTHER SHOPS IN THE CAMP THAT ARE OFFERING THE SAME SERVICE.
BUT WE ARE BY FAR THE BEST. THE OTHER GUYS DON'T HAVE A CLUE ABOUT MUSIC.
DYNACORD POWERMATE 1600 (MADE IN GERMANY!)
PMP01500W SUPER KARAOKE ACTIVE STEREO SPEAKER WITH BUILT-IN AMPLIFIER

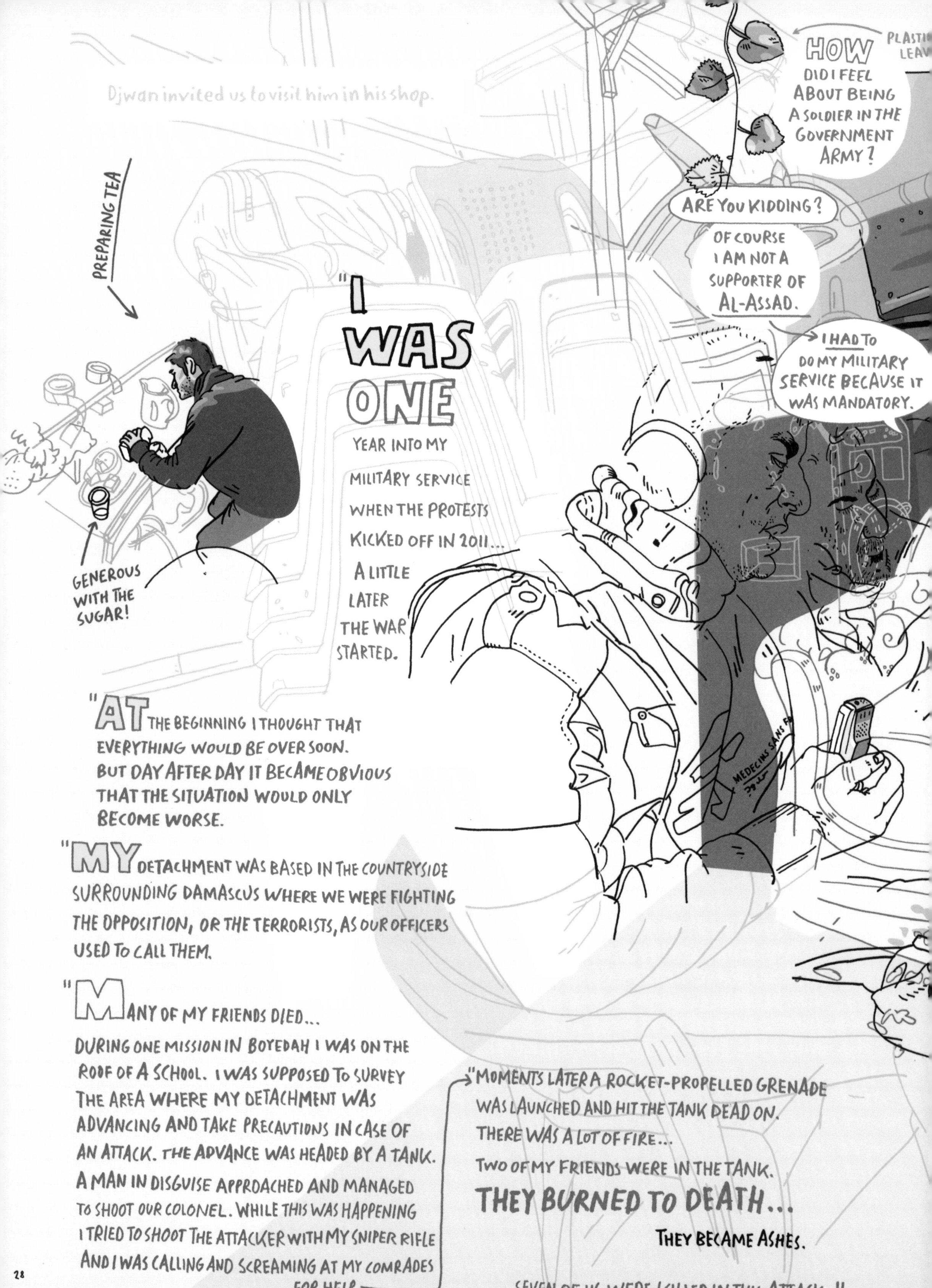
Djwan invited us to visit him in his shop.
PREPARING TEA
GENEROUS WITH THE SUGAR!
"I WAS ONE YEAR INTO MY MILITARY SERVICE WHEN THE PROTESTS KICKED OFF IN 2011... A LITTLE LATER THE WAR STARTED.
HOW DID I FEEL ABOUT BEING A SOLDIER IN THE GOVERNMENT ARMY?
ARE YOU KIDDING?
OF COURSE I AM NOT A SUPPORTER OF AL-ASSAD.
I HAD TO DO MY MILITARY SERVICE BECAUSE IT WAS MANDATORY.
MEDECINS SANS F
"AT THE BEGINNING I THOUGHT THAT EVERYTHING WOULD BE OVER SOON. BUT DAY AFTER DAY IT BECAME OBVIOUS THAT THE SITUATION WOULD ONLY BECOME WORSE.
"MY DETACHMENT WAS BASED IN THE COUNTRYSIDE SURROUNDING DAMASCUS WHERE WE WERE FIGHTING THE OPPOSITION, OR THE TERRORISTS, AS OUR OFFICERS USED TO CALL THEM.
"MANY OF MY FRIENDS DIED...
DURING ONE MISSION IN BOYEDAH I WAS ON THE ROOF OF A SCHOOL. I WAS SUPPOSED TO SURVEY THE AREA WHERE MY DETACHMENT WAS ADVANCING AND TAKE PRECAUTIONS IN CASE OF AN ATTACK. THE ADVANCE WAS HEADED BY A TANK. A MAN IN DISGUISE APPROACHED AND MANAGED TO SHOOT OUR COLONEL. WHILE THIS WAS HAPPENING I TRIED TO SHOOT THE ATTACKER WITH MY SNIPER RIFLE AND I WAS CALLING AND SCREAMING AT MY COMRADES FOR HELP.
"MOMENTS LATER A ROCKET-PROPELLED GRENADE WAS LAUNCHED AND HIT THE TANK DEAD ON.
THERE WAS A LOT OF FIRE...
TWO OF MY FRIENDS WERE IN THE TANK.
THEY BURNED TO DEATH...
THEY BECAME ASHES.
SEVEN OF US WERE KILLED IN THIS ATTACK..."

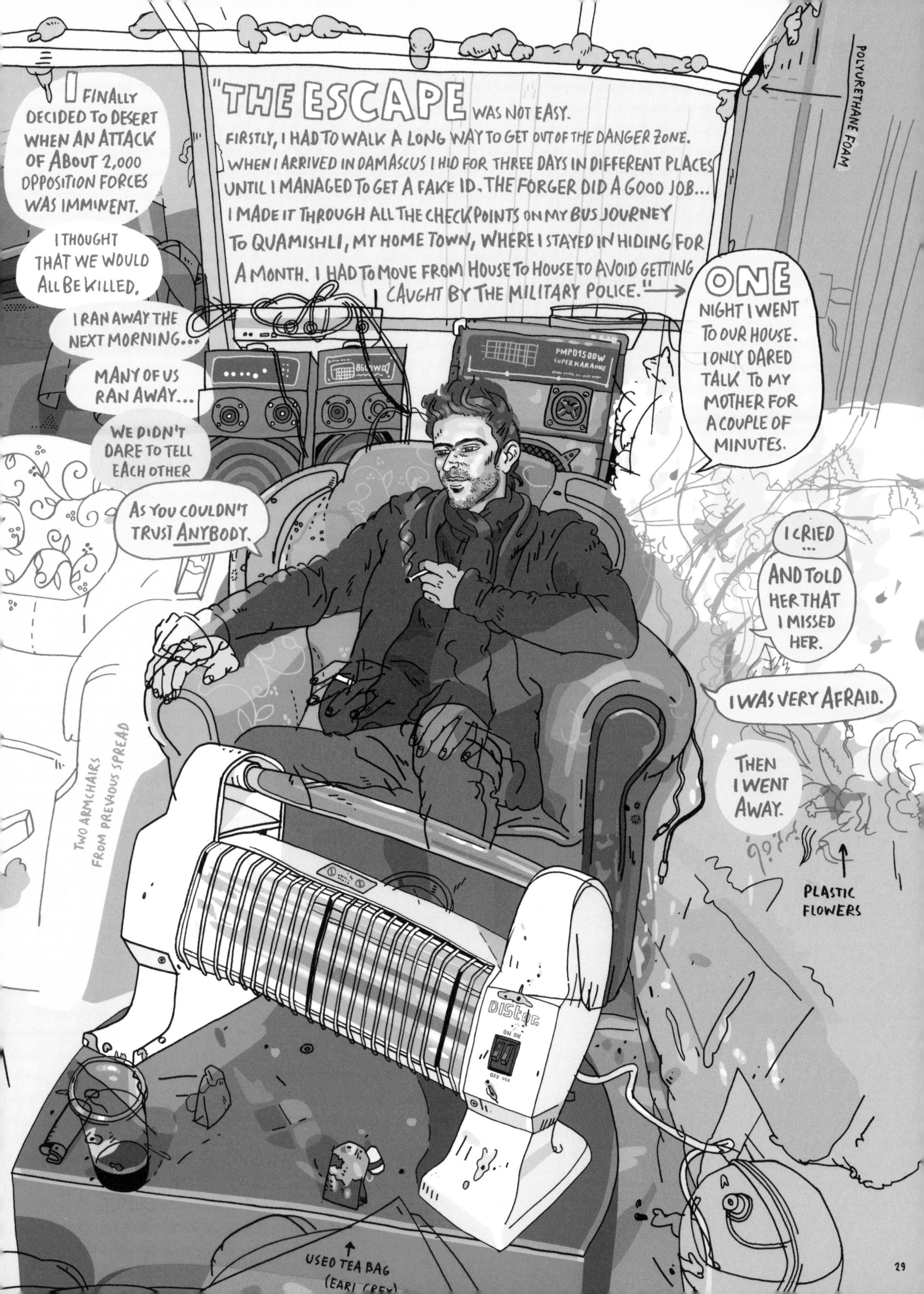
I FINALLY DECIDED TO DESERT WHEN AN ATTACK OF ABOUT 2,000 OPPOSITION FORCES WAS IMMINENT.
I THOUGHT THAT WE WOULD ALL BE KILLED.
I RAN AWAY THE NEXT MORNING...
MANY OF US RAN AWAY...
WE DIDN'T DARE TO TELL EACH OTHER
AS YOU COULDN'T TRUST ANYBODY.
"THE ESCAPE WAS NOT EASY.
FIRSTLY, I HAD TO WALK A LONG WAY TO GET OUT OF THE DANGER ZONE.
WHEN I ARRIVED IN DAMASCUS I HID FOR THREE DAYS IN DIFFERENT PLACES
UNTIL I MANAGED TO GET A FAKE ID. THE FORGER DID A GOOD JOB...
I MADE IT THROUGH ALL THE CHECKPOINTS ON MY BUS JOURNEY
TO QUAMISHLI, MY HOME TOWN, WHERE I STAYED IN HIDING FOR
A MONTH. I HAD TO MOVE FROM HOUSE TO HOUSE TO AVOID GETTING
CAUGHT BY THE MILITARY POLICE."
ONE NIGHT I WENT TO OUR HOUSE. I ONLY DARED TALK TO MY MOTHER FOR A COUPLE OF MINUTES.
I CRIED ...
AND TOLD HER THAT I MISSED HER.
I WAS VERY AFRAID.
THEN I WENT AWAY.
POLYURETHANE FOAM
TWO ARMCHAIRS FROM PREVIOUS SPREAD
PLASTIC FLOWERS
USED TEA BAG
(EARL GREY)

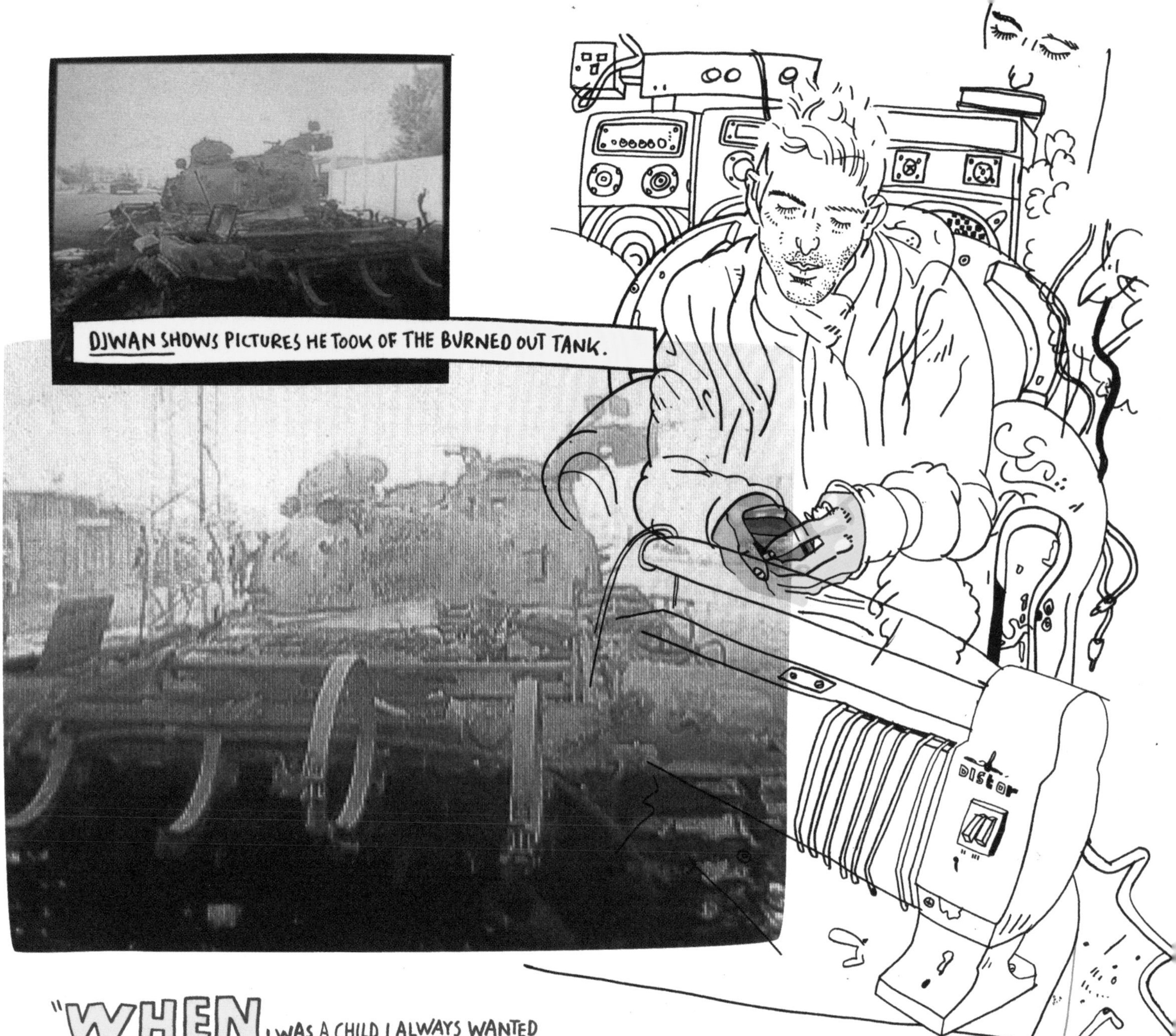
DJWAN SHOWS PICTURES HE TOOK OF THE BURNED OUT TANK.
DISTOR

"WHEN I WAS A CHILD I ALWAYS WANTED TO BECOME A TEACHER... THIS WAS MY DREAM. IT DIDN'T MATTER TO ME WHAT KIND OF TEACHER... JUST BECOMING ANY KIND OF TEACHER SEEMED TO BE FINE TO ME. WHEN I WAS 16 I STARTED HELPING OUT IN MY UNCLE'S BUTCHER SHOP, WHEN I CAME BACK FROM HIGH SCHOOL IN THE AFTERNOON. I HATED IT BECAUSE OF THE ANIMALS' BLOOD. IT WAS DISGUSTING! I WORKED THERE UNTIL I WENT TO LEBANON.

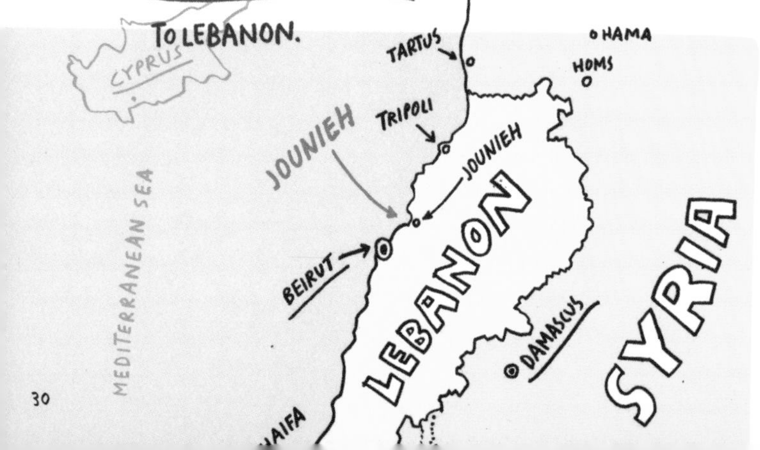
CYPRUS
TARTUS
HAMA
HOMS
TRIPOLI
JOUNIEH
JOUNIEH
MEDITERRANEAN SEA
BEIRUT
LEBANON
DAMASCUS
SYRIA
HAIFA

"I WAS 19 WHEN I WENT TO JONIEH, LEBANON, TO WORK THERE AS A WAITER IN A BAR. I WENT THERE LIKE EVERYBODY ELSE, TO SAVE SOME MONEY IN ORDER TO GET ME THROUGH MY MILITARY SERVICE. BECAUSE YOU WILL DIE OF HUNGER IF YOU RELY ON THE ARMY LOOKING AFTER YOU. (DJWAN LAUGHS A LOT AFTER HE SAYS THIS.) I DIDN'T HAVE A GOOD TIME IN JONIEH. EVEN THOUGH THE TOWN IS A BEAUTIFUL AND POPULAR MEDITERRANEAN RESORT... I HAD TO WORK LONG HOURS. IT WAS EXHAUSTING AND I COULD HARDLY FIND THE TIME TO DO ANYTHING FUN.

"SEVERAL MONTHS AFTER MY ARRIVAL IN LEBANON MY FATHER PASSED AWAY. I WANTED TO GO AND SEE HIS BODY AND ATTEND THE FUNERAL BUT AS SOON AS I CROSSED THE BORDER INTO SYRIA I WAS ARRESTED BY THE MILITARY POLICE. I WAS IMMEDIATELY DRAFTED INTO THE ARMY AND WASN'T ABLE TO SEE MY FATHER'S BODY...

"WE HAVE TO START OUR MILITARY SERVICE AT THE AGE OF 18... I JOINED LATE. WHEN YOU SHOW UP LATE THE MILITARY POLICE WILL DEFINITELY CAPTURE YOU AS EVERYBODY KNOWS... EVEN IF YOU ARE HIDING ON THE MOON!

"BEFORE EVERY NEW MISSION OUR COMMANDING OFFICER TOLD US: 'EVERYTHING IS FINE. DON'T BE SCARED. YOU ARE HERE TO FIGHT FOR YOUR PEOPLE.'

WAS I SCARED?

NO ONE CAN SAY: 'I AM A MAN AND THEREFORE I AM NOT AFRAID.' WE WERE ALL SCARED. YOU HOPE TO SURVIVE ONE MISSION. WHEN THE MISSION IS OVER ANOTHER ONE COMES AND YOU ARE AWARE THAT YOU COULD GET KILLED AT ANY GIVEN MOMENT.

"HOW DID I BECOME A SNIPER? I BECAME A SNIPER BY DRAWING LOTS... AT THE BEGINNING OF MILITARY SERVICE THEY USUALLY DECIDE WHAT EACH RECRUIT WILL DO AT RANDOM.

WHAT I LIKED ABOUT THE ARMY WAS THE CAMARADERIE... I MADE VERY GOOD FRIENDS.

"ONE OF MY FRIENDS SHOT HIMSELF WITH HIS RIFLE. THREE BULLETS... TWO OF THEM PENETRATED HIS BODY AND THE THIRD ONE WENT INTO THE AIR. MY COMMANDER PUT ME IN JAIL BECAUSE OF THAT. WE USED TO LIVE IN THE SAME TENT AND THE COMMANDER ACCUSED ME OF KILLING MY FRIEND.

"I DON'T KNOW WHY HE KILLED HIMSELF EXACTLY... IT MUST HAVE BEEN AN ACCUMULATION OF EVENTS. HIS FATHER HAD ALREADY BEEN DEAD FOR A LONG TIME AND HIS MOTHER HAD DIED RECENTLY... THE COMMANDER DID NOT LET HIM ATTEND HER FUNERAL. ON TOP OF THAT HIS BROTHER WAS MURDERED. SINCE THEN HIS SISTER HAD BEEN SUFFERING FROM DEPRESSION. A COUPLE OF DAYS BEFORE MY FRIEND KILLED HIMSELF HE RECEIVED A PHONE CALL FROM HIS UNCLE WHO TOLD HIM THAT HIS SISTER HAD GONE OUT INTO THE STREET AND STARTED SCREAMING UNCONTROLLABLY... THAT SHE HAD BECOME COMPLETELY CRAZY.

"SO MY COMMANDING OFFICERS STARTED AN INVESTIGATION INCLUDING A LOT OF INTERROGATION AND TORTURE. THEY HUNG ME FROM THE PRISON'S CEILING AND BEAT ME. THEY WHIP YOU AND ELECTROCUTE YOU UNTIL YOU CONFESS TO SOMETHING YOU DIDN'T DO. THEY ALSO KEPT ON INSULTING ME AND SAID TERRIBLE THINGS ABOUT MEMBERS OF MY FAMILY. OF COURSE THE FOOD WAS DISGUSTING AND THE PORTIONS WERE SMALL. I WAS ALWAYS HUNGRY. AFTER A WEEK THEY REALIZED I HAD NOT KILLED MY FRIEND.

"WHEN I ARRIVED IN DOMIZ I FELT VERY SAD... I WAS ALLOCATED A SPACE IN A TENT WITH FIVE OTHER GUYS. THE TENT IS LOCATED IN THE CAMP'S SINGLE MEN'S AREA. THE LIVING CONDITIONS THERE ARE BAD. THERE IS ALWAYS A SHORTAGE OF WATER... WE HAVE THE FEELING THAT WE ARE BEING NEGLECTED BY EVERYONE."

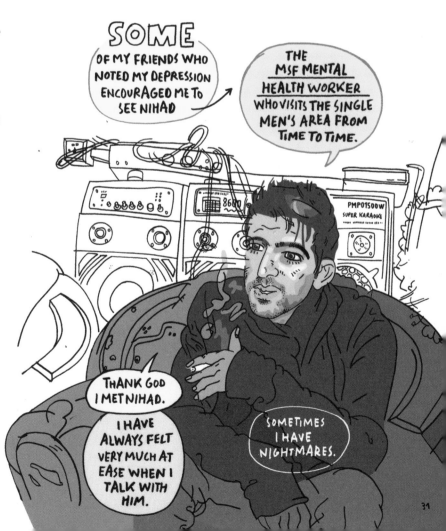

SOME OF MY FRIENDS WHO NOTED MY DEPRESSION ENCOURAGED ME TO SEE NIHAD

THE MSF MENTAL HEALTH WORKER WHO VISITS THE SINGLE MEN'S AREA FROM TIME TO TIME.

THANK GOD I MET NIHAD.

I HAVE ALWAYS FELT VERY MUCH AT EASE WHEN I TALK WITH HIM.

SOMETIMES I HAVE NIGHTMARES.

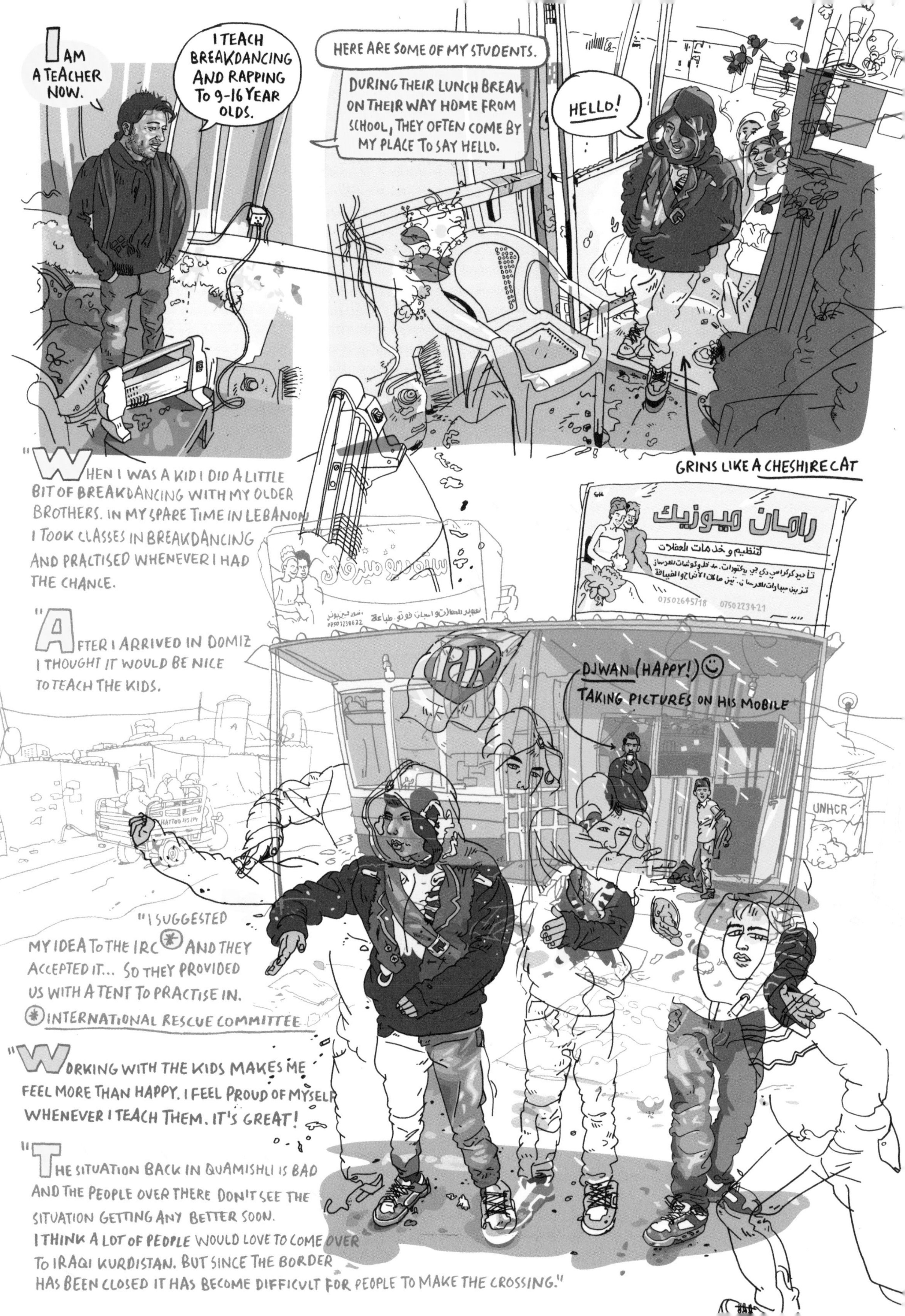
I AM A TEACHER NOW.
I TEACH BREAKDANCING AND RAPPING TO 9-16 YEAR OLDS.
HERE ARE SOME OF MY STUDENTS.
DURING THEIR LUNCH BREAK, ON THEIR WAY HOME FROM SCHOOL, THEY OFTEN COME BY MY PLACE TO SAY HELLO.
HELLO!
GRINS LIKE A CHESHIRE CAT
"WHEN I WAS A KID I DID A LITTLE BIT OF BREAKDANCING WITH MY OLDER BROTHERS. IN MY SPARE TIME IN LEBANON I TOOK CLASSES IN BREAKDANCING AND PRACTISED WHENEVER I HAD THE CHANCE.
رامان ميوزيك
تنظيم وخدمات الحفلات
"AFTER I ARRIVED IN DOMIZ I THOUGHT IT WOULD BE NICE TO TEACH THE KIDS.
DJWAN (HAPPY!) ☺ TAKING PICTURES ON HIS MOBILE
UNHCR
"I SUGGESTED MY IDEA TO THE IRC * AND THEY ACCEPTED IT... SO THEY PROVIDED US WITH A TENT TO PRACTISE IN.
* INTERNATIONAL RESCUE COMMITTEE
"WORKING WITH THE KIDS MAKES ME FEEL MORE THAN HAPPY. I FEEL PROUD OF MYSELF WHENEVER I TEACH THEM. IT'S GREAT!
"THE SITUATION BACK IN QUAMISHLI IS BAD AND THE PEOPLE OVER THERE DON'T SEE THE SITUATION GETTING ANY BETTER SOON.
I THINK A LOT OF PEOPLE WOULD LOVE TO COME OVER TO IRAQI KURDISTAN. BUT SINCE THE BORDER HAS BEEN CLOSED IT HAS BECOME DIFFICULT FOR PEOPLE TO MAKE THE CROSSING."

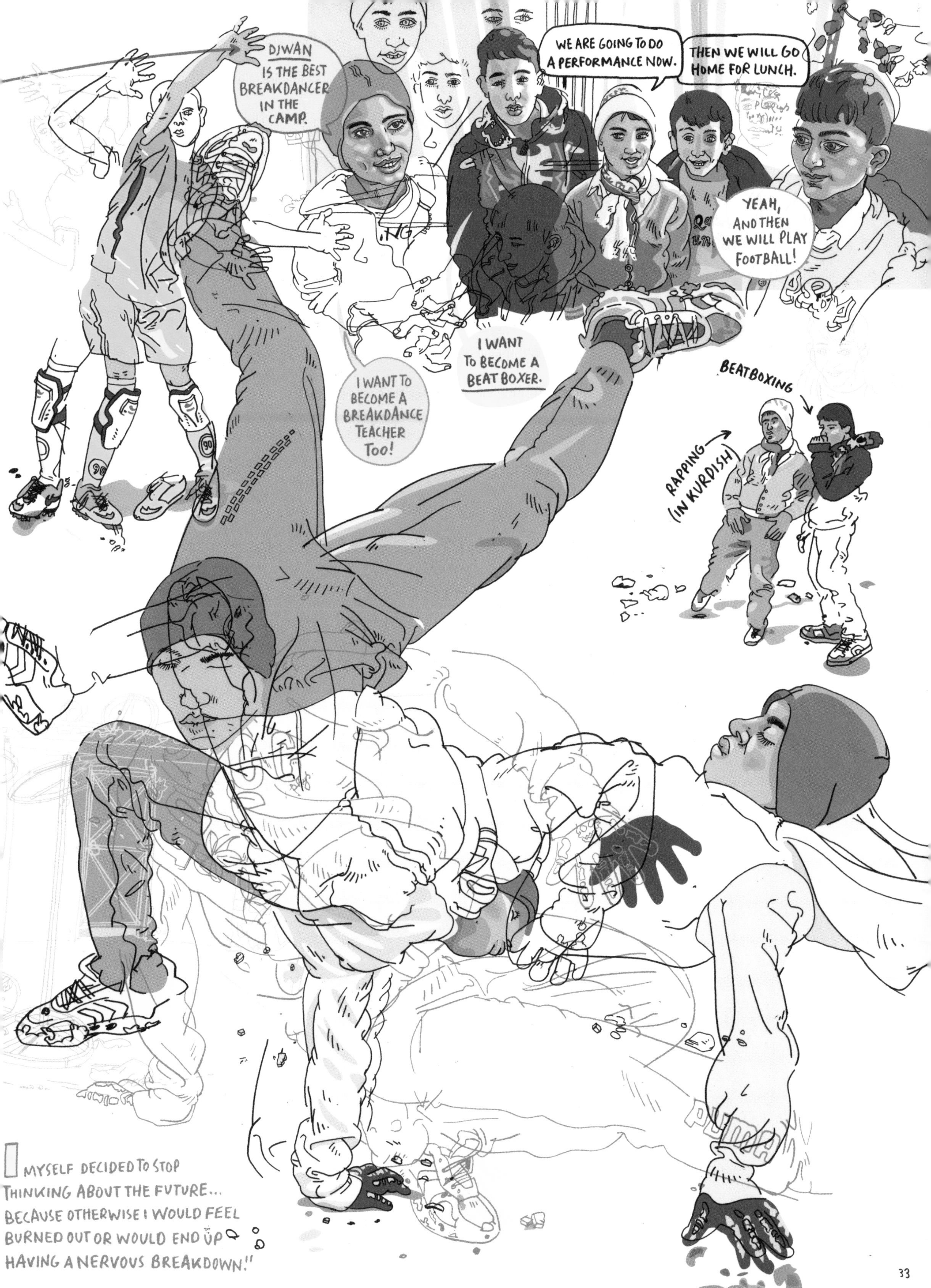
DJWAN IS THE BEST BREAKDANCER IN THE CAMP.
WE ARE GOING TO DO A PERFORMANCE NOW.
THEN WE WILL GO HOME FOR LUNCH.
YEAH, AND THEN WE WILL PLAY FOOTBALL!
I WANT TO BECOME A BEAT BOXER.
I WANT TO BECOME A BREAKDANCE TEACHER TOO!
BEATBOXING
RAPPING (IN KURDISH)
I MYSELF DECIDED TO STOP THINKING ABOUT THE FUTURE... BECAUSE OTHERWISE I WOULD FEEL BURNED OUT OR WOULD END UP HAVING A NERVOUS BREAKDOWN."

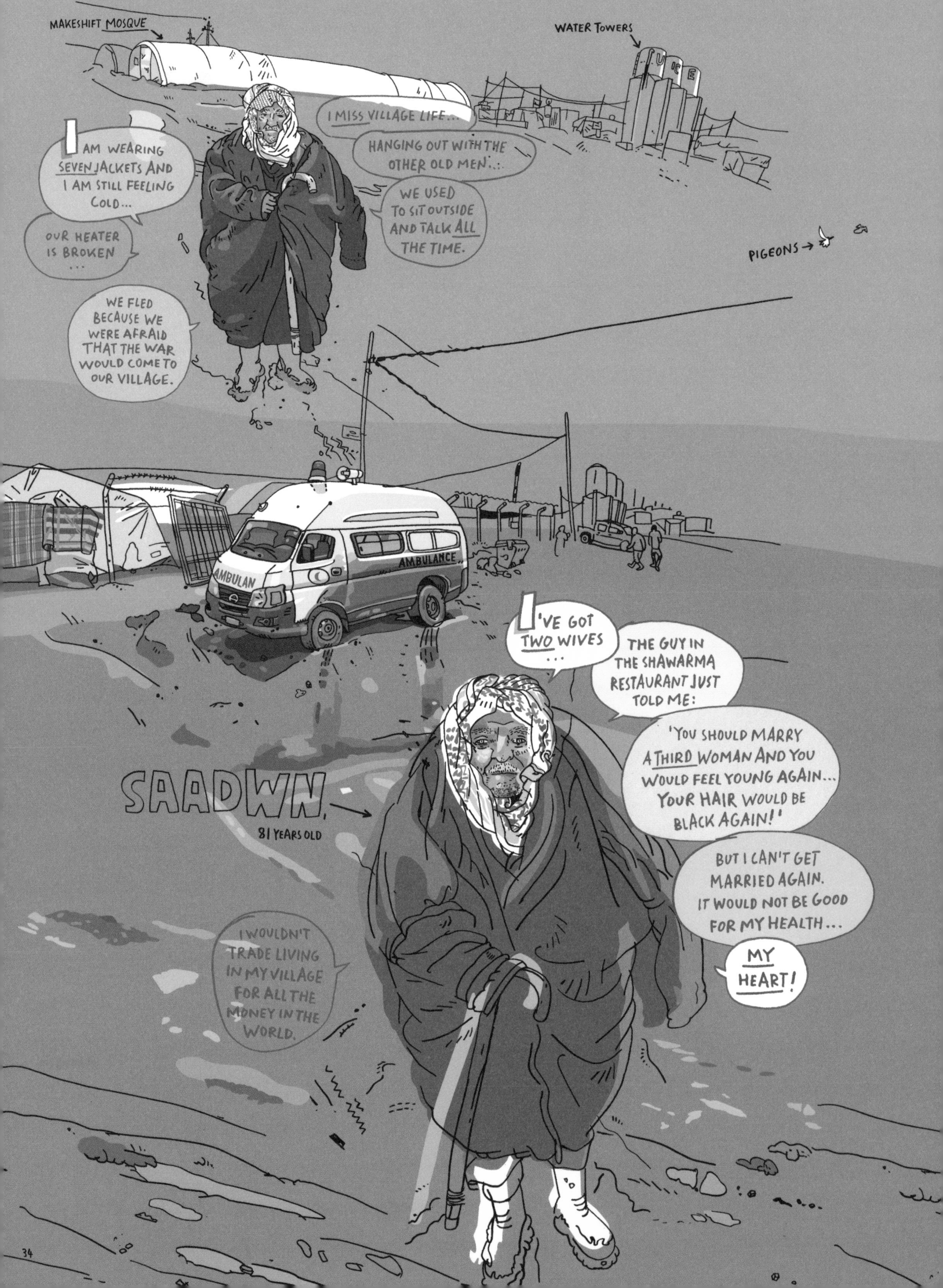
MAKESHIFT MOSQUE
WATER TOWERS
I AM WEARING SEVEN JACKETS AND I AM STILL FEELING COLD...
OUR HEATER IS BROKEN ...
I MISS VILLAGE LIFE...
HANGING OUT WITH THE OTHER OLD MEN...
WE USED TO SIT OUTSIDE AND TALK ALL THE TIME.
PIGEONS
WE FLED BECAUSE WE WERE AFRAID THAT THE WAR WOULD COME TO OUR VILLAGE.
AMBULAN
AMBULANCE
SAADWN,
81 YEARS OLD
I'VE GOT TWO WIVES ...
THE GUY IN THE SHAWARMA RESTAURANT JUST TOLD ME:
'YOU SHOULD MARRY A THIRD WOMAN AND YOU WOULD FEEL YOUNG AGAIN... YOUR HAIR WOULD BE BLACK AGAIN!'
BUT I CAN'T GET MARRIED AGAIN. IT WOULD NOT BE GOOD FOR MY HEALTH...
MY HEART!
I WOULDN'T TRADE LIVING IN MY VILLAGE FOR ALL THE MONEY IN THE WORLD.

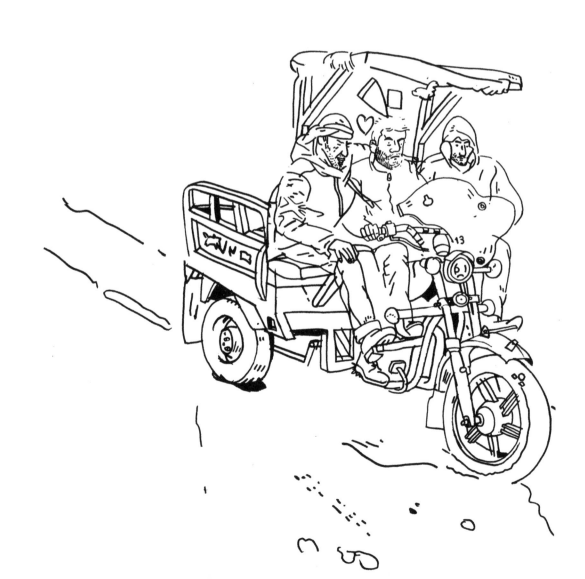

GREECE

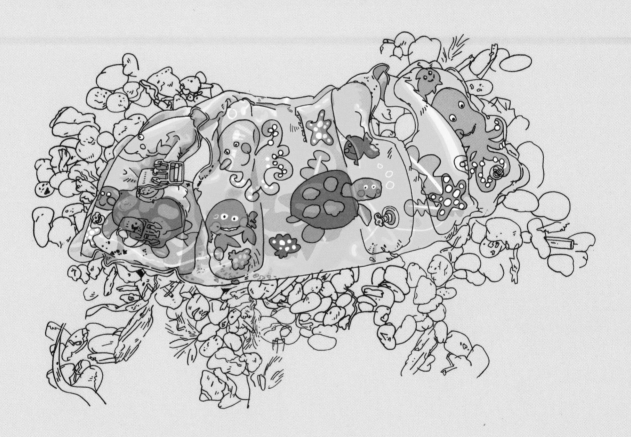

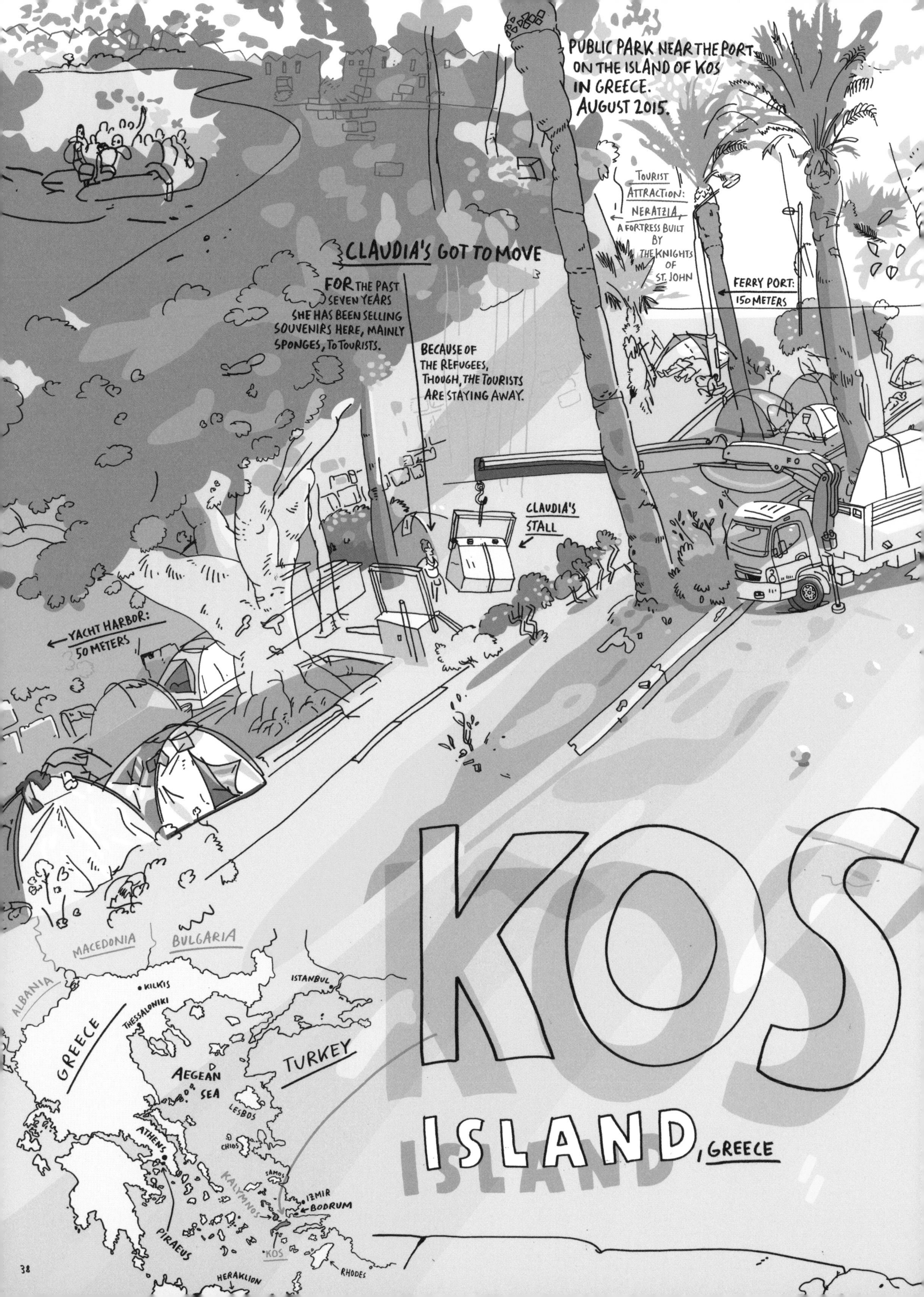

PUBLIC PARK NEAR THE PORT ON THE ISLAND OF KOS IN GREECE. AUGUST 2015.
TOURIST ATTRACTION: NERATZIA, A FORTRESS BUILT BY THE KNIGHTS OF ST. JOHN
CLAUDIA'S GOT TO MOVE
FOR THE PAST SEVEN YEARS SHE HAS BEEN SELLING SOUVENIRS HERE, MAINLY SPONGES, TO TOURISTS.
BECAUSE OF THE REFUGEES, THOUGH, THE TOURISTS ARE STAYING AWAY.
FERRY PORT: 150 METERS
CLAUDIA'S STALL
YACHT HARBOR: 50 METERS
KOS
ISLAND, GREECE
MACEDONIA
BULGARIA
ALBANIA
KILKIS
ISTANBUL
THESSALONIKI
GREECE
TURKEY
AEGEAN SEA
LESBOS
ATHENS
CHIOS
SAMOS
KALYMNOS
IZMIR
BODRUM
PIRAEUS
KOS
RHODES
HERAKLION

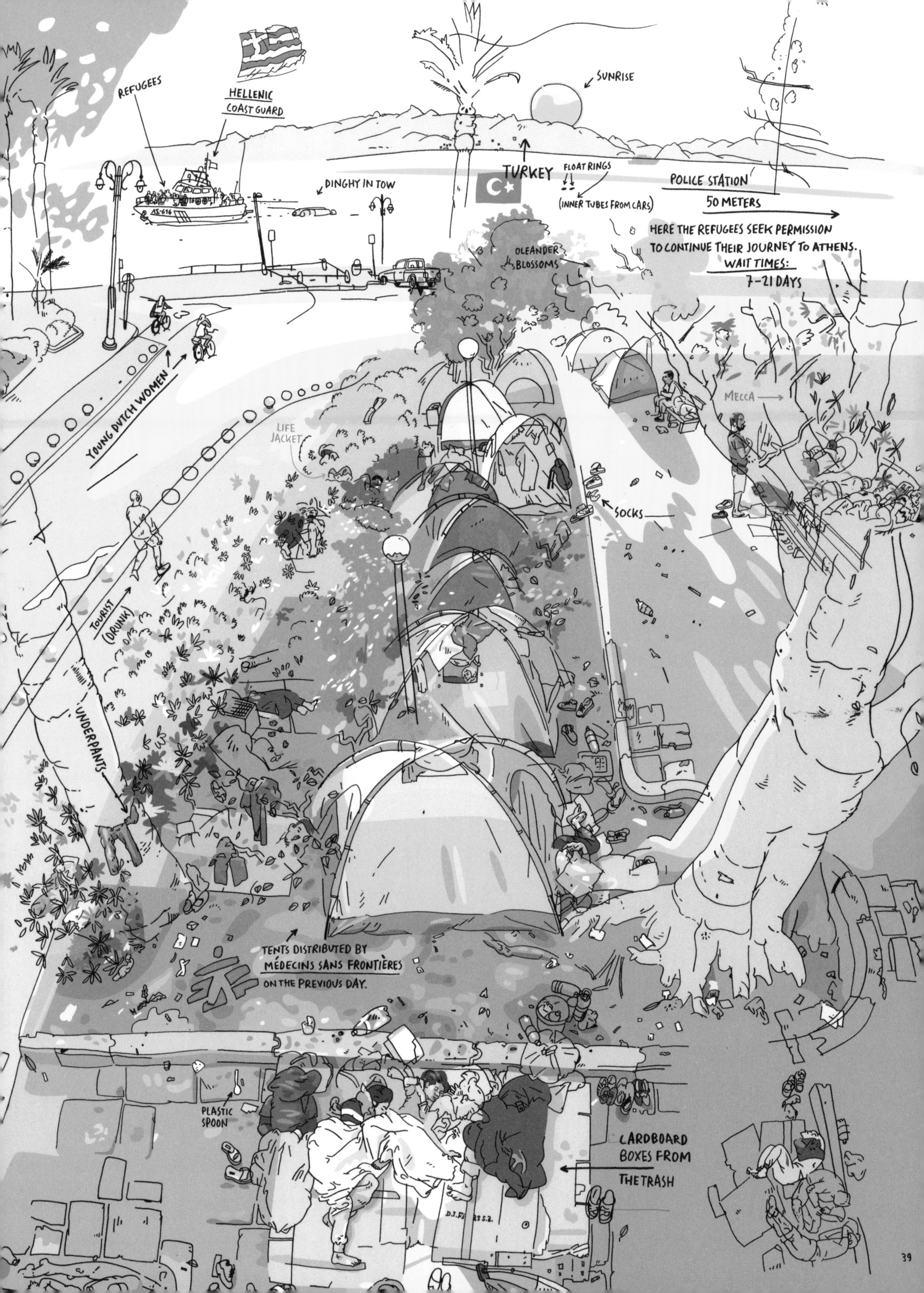
REFUGEES
HELLENIC COAST GUARD
SUNRISE
DINGHY IN TOW
TURKEY
FLOAT RINGS
(INNER TUBES FROM CARS)
POLICE STATION
50 METERS
HERE THE REFUGEES SEEK PERMISSION TO CONTINUE THEIR JOURNEY TO ATHENS.
WAIT TIMES:
7–21 DAYS
OLEANDER BLOSSOMS
MECCA
YOUNG DUTCH WOMEN
LIFE JACKET
SOCKS
TOURIST (DRUNK)
UNDERPANTS
TENTS DISTRIBUTED BY MÉDECINS SANS FRONTIÈRES ON THE PREVIOUS DAY.
PLASTIC SPOON
CARDBOARD BOXES FROM THE TRASH

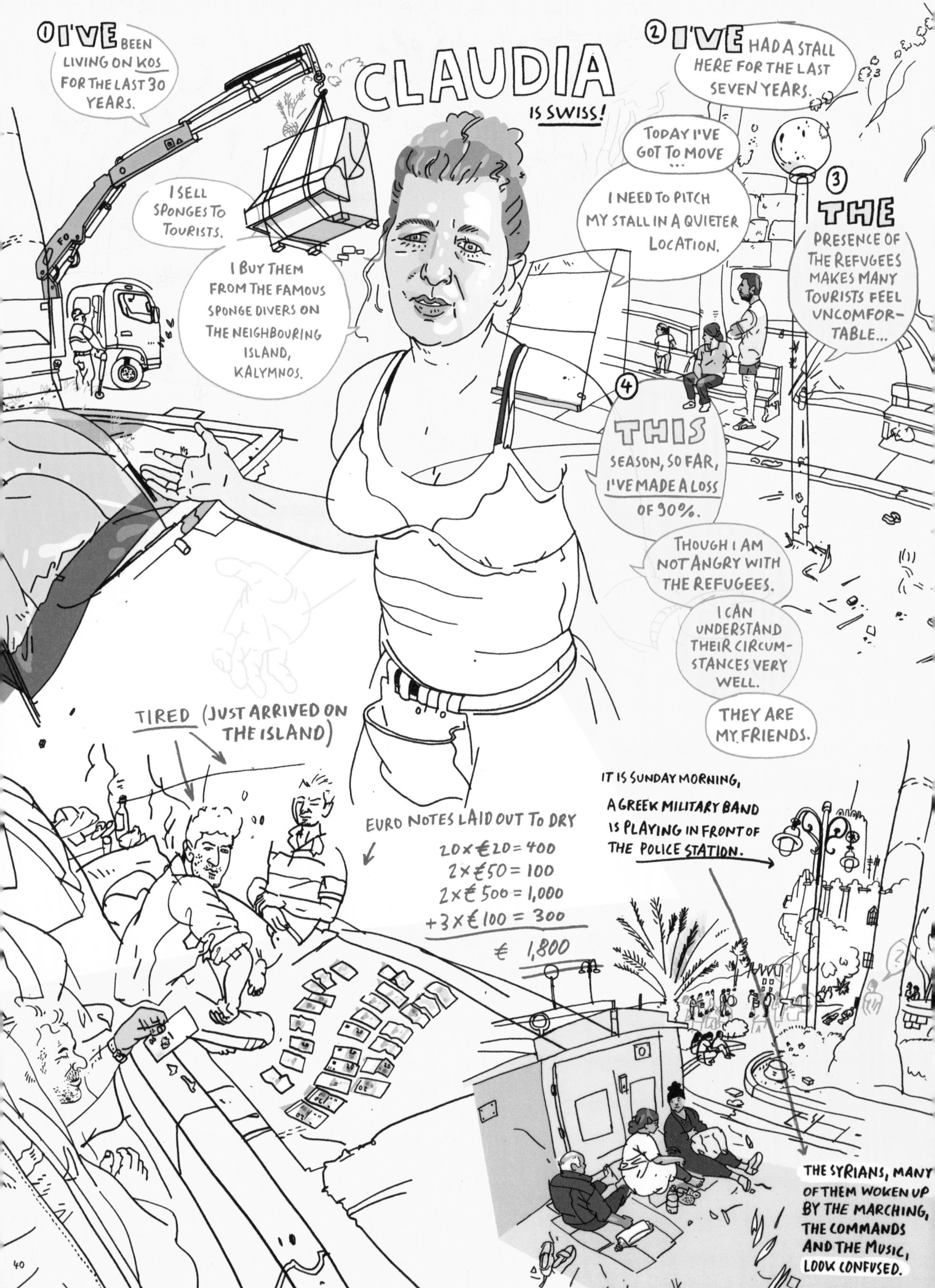

CLAUDIA
IS SWISS!
1 I'VE BEEN LIVING ON KOS FOR THE LAST 30 YEARS.
I SELL SPONGES TO TOURISTS.
I BUY THEM FROM THE FAMOUS SPONGE DIVERS ON THE NEIGHBOURING ISLAND, KALYMNOS.
2 I'VE HAD A STALL HERE FOR THE LAST SEVEN YEARS.
TODAY I'VE GOT TO MOVE ...
I NEED TO PITCH MY STALL IN A QUIETER LOCATION.
3 THE PRESENCE OF THE REFUGEES MAKES MANY TOURISTS FEEL UNCOMFORTABLE...
4 THIS SEASON, SO FAR, I'VE MADE A LOSS OF 90%.
THOUGH I AM NOT ANGRY WITH THE REFUGEES.
I CAN UNDERSTAND THEIR CIRCUMSTANCES VERY WELL.
THEY ARE MY FRIENDS.
TIRED (JUST ARRIVED ON THE ISLAND)
EURO NOTES LAID OUT TO DRY
20×€20 = 400
2×€50 = 100
2×€500 = 1,000
+3×€100 = 300
€ 1,800
IT IS SUNDAY MORNING, A GREEK MILITARY BAND IS PLAYING IN FRONT OF THE POLICE STATION.
THE SYRIANS, MANY OF THEM WOKEN UP BY THE MARCHING, THE COMMANDS AND THE MUSIC, LOOK CONFUSED.

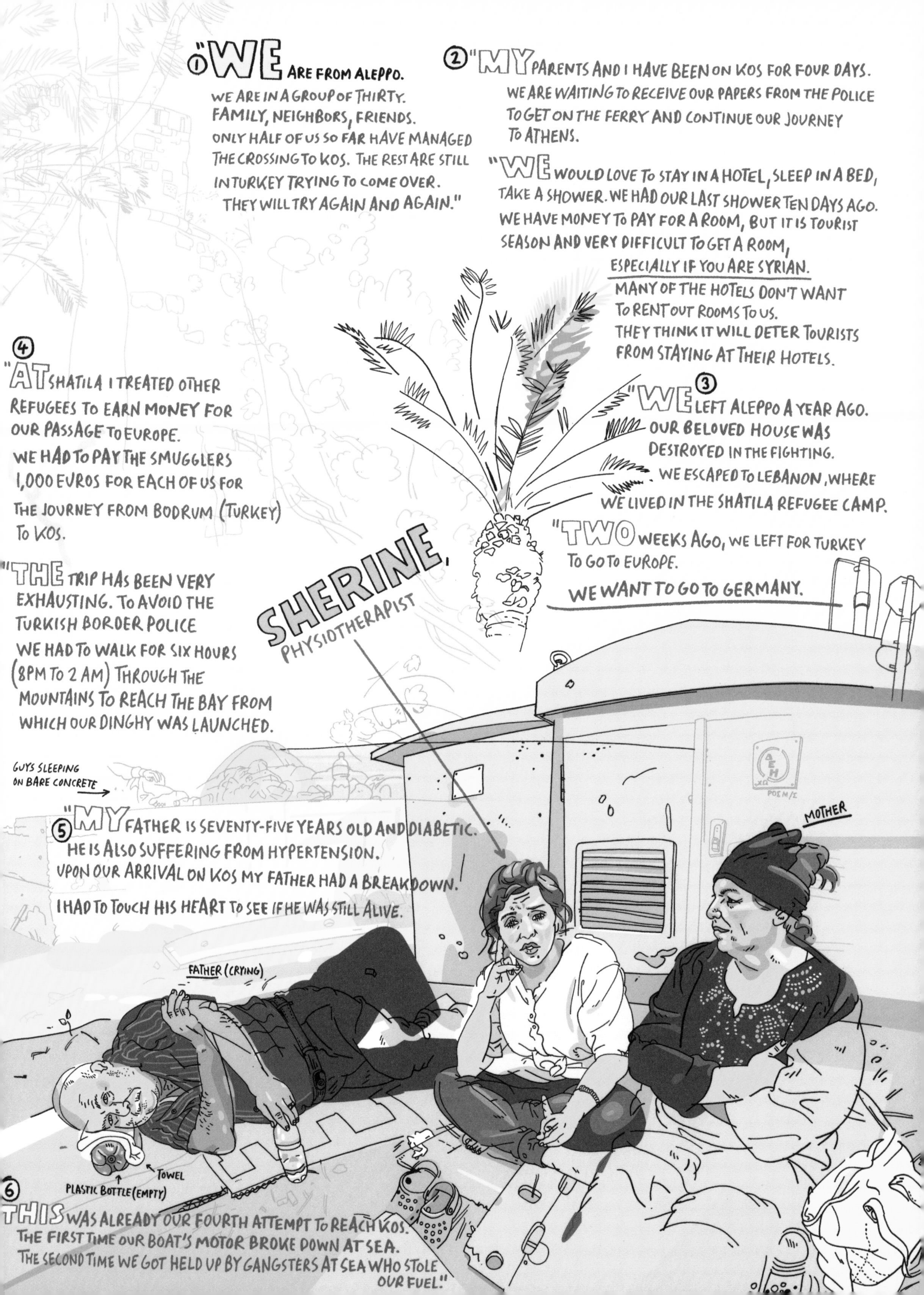

① "WE ARE FROM ALEPPO.
WE ARE IN A GROUP OF THIRTY.
FAMILY, NEIGHBORS, FRIENDS.
ONLY HALF OF US SO FAR HAVE MANAGED THE CROSSING TO KOS. THE REST ARE STILL IN TURKEY TRYING TO COME OVER.
THEY WILL TRY AGAIN AND AGAIN."
② "MY PARENTS AND I HAVE BEEN ON KOS FOR FOUR DAYS.
WE ARE WAITING TO RECEIVE OUR PAPERS FROM THE POLICE TO GET ON THE FERRY AND CONTINUE OUR JOURNEY TO ATHENS.
"WE WOULD LOVE TO STAY IN A HOTEL, SLEEP IN A BED, TAKE A SHOWER. WE HAD OUR LAST SHOWER TEN DAYS AGO. WE HAVE MONEY TO PAY FOR A ROOM, BUT IT IS TOURIST SEASON AND VERY DIFFICULT TO GET A ROOM,
ESPECIALLY IF YOU ARE SYRIAN.
MANY OF THE HOTELS DON'T WANT TO RENT OUT ROOMS TO US.
THEY THINK IT WILL DETER TOURISTS FROM STAYING AT THEIR HOTELS.
③ "WE LEFT ALEPPO A YEAR AGO.
OUR BELOVED HOUSE WAS DESTROYED IN THE FIGHTING.
WE ESCAPED TO LEBANON, WHERE WE LIVED IN THE SHATILA REFUGEE CAMP.
"TWO WEEKS AGO, WE LEFT FOR TURKEY TO GO TO EUROPE.
WE WANT TO GO TO GERMANY.
④ "AT SHATILA I TREATED OTHER REFUGEES TO EARN MONEY FOR OUR PASSAGE TO EUROPE.
WE HAD TO PAY THE SMUGGLERS 1,000 EUROS FOR EACH OF US FOR THE JOURNEY FROM BODRUM (TURKEY) TO KOS.
"THE TRIP HAS BEEN VERY EXHAUSTING. TO AVOID THE TURKISH BORDER POLICE
WE HAD TO WALK FOR SIX HOURS (8PM TO 2 AM) THROUGH THE MOUNTAINS TO REACH THE BAY FROM WHICH OUR DINGHY WAS LAUNCHED.
SHERINE,
PHYSIOTHERAPIST
GUYS SLEEPING ON BARE CONCRETE
⑤ "MY FATHER IS SEVENTY-FIVE YEARS OLD AND DIABETIC.
HE IS ALSO SUFFERING FROM HYPERTENSION.
UPON OUR ARRIVAL ON KOS MY FATHER HAD A BREAKDOWN.
I HAD TO TOUCH HIS HEART TO SEE IF HE WAS STILL ALIVE.
MOTHER
FATHER (CRYING)
TOWEL
PLASTIC BOTTLE (EMPTY)
⑥ THIS WAS ALREADY OUR FOURTH ATTEMPT TO REACH KOS.
THE FIRST TIME OUR BOAT'S MOTOR BROKE DOWN AT SEA.
THE SECOND TIME WE GOT HELD UP BY GANGSTERS AT SEA WHO STOLE OUR FUEL."

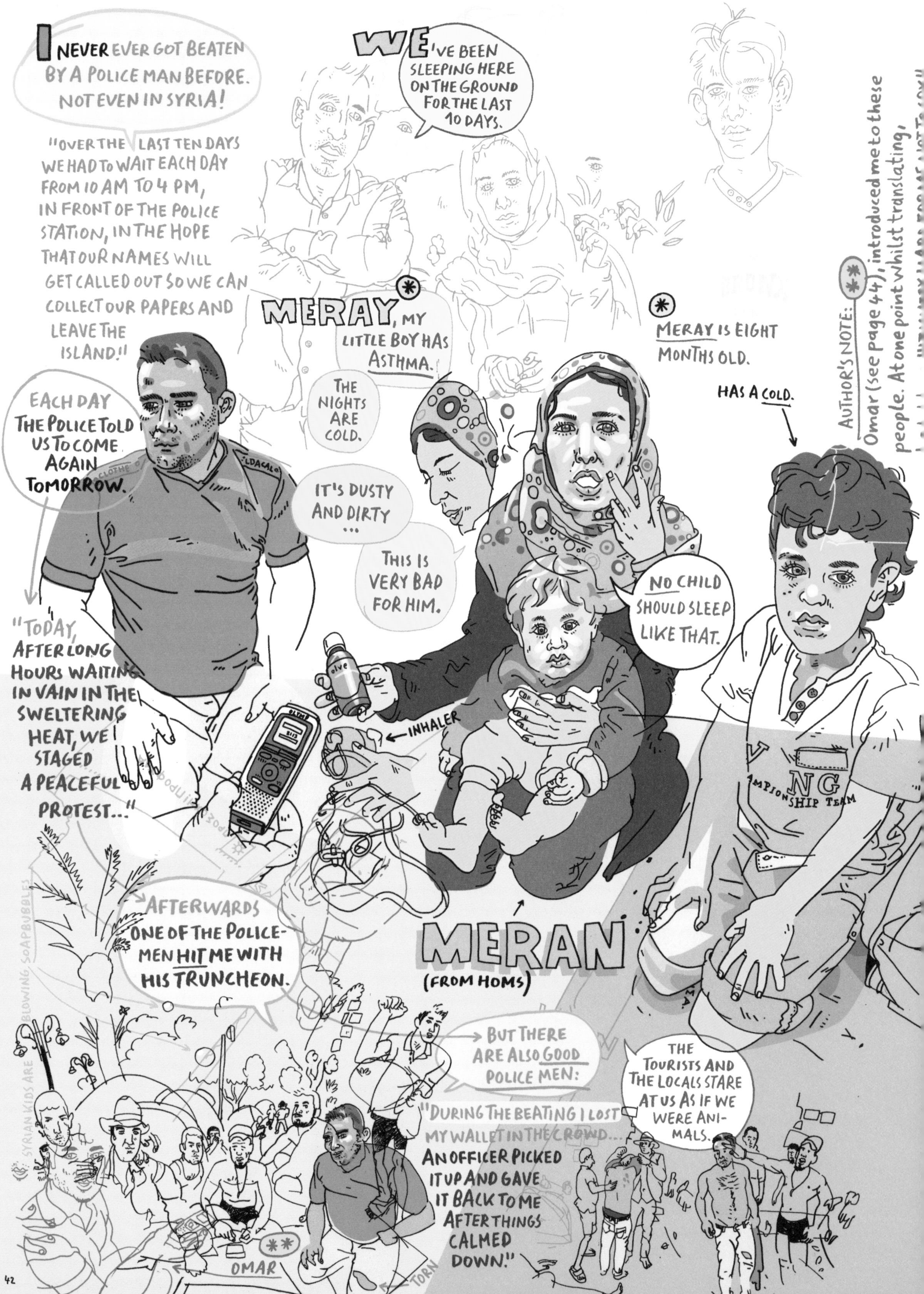
I NEVER EVER GOT BEATEN BY A POLICE MAN BEFORE. NOT EVEN IN SYRIA!
"OVER THE LAST TEN DAYS WE HAD TO WAIT EACH DAY FROM 10 AM TO 4 PM, IN FRONT OF THE POLICE STATION, IN THE HOPE THAT OUR NAMES WILL GET CALLED OUT SO WE CAN COLLECT OUR PAPERS AND LEAVE THE ISLAND!"
WE'VE BEEN SLEEPING HERE ON THE GROUND FOR THE LAST 10 DAYS.
MERAY*, MY LITTLE BOY HAS ASTHMA.
THE NIGHTS ARE COLD.
IT'S DUSTY AND DIRTY ...
THIS IS VERY BAD FOR HIM.
* MERAY IS EIGHT MONTHS OLD.
HAS A COLD.
NO CHILD SHOULD SLEEP LIKE THAT.
AUTHOR'S NOTE: ** Omar (see page 44), introduced me to these people. At one point whilst translating,
EACH DAY THE POLICE TOLD US TO COME AGAIN TOMORROW.
"TODAY, AFTER LONG HOURS WAITING IN VAIN IN THE SWELTERING HEAT, WE STAGED A PEACEFUL PROTEST..."
INHALER
MERAN
(FROM HOMS)
AFTERWARDS ONE OF THE POLICE-MEN HIT ME WITH HIS TRUNCHEON.
BUT THERE ARE ALSO GOOD POLICE MEN:
"DURING THE BEATING I LOST MY WALLET IN THE CROWD... AN OFFICER PICKED IT UP AND GAVE IT BACK TO ME AFTER THINGS CALMED DOWN."
THE TOURISTS AND THE LOCALS STARE AT US AS IF WE WERE ANI-MALS.
SYRIAN KIDS ARE BLOWING SOAPBUBBLES
** OMAR
TORN

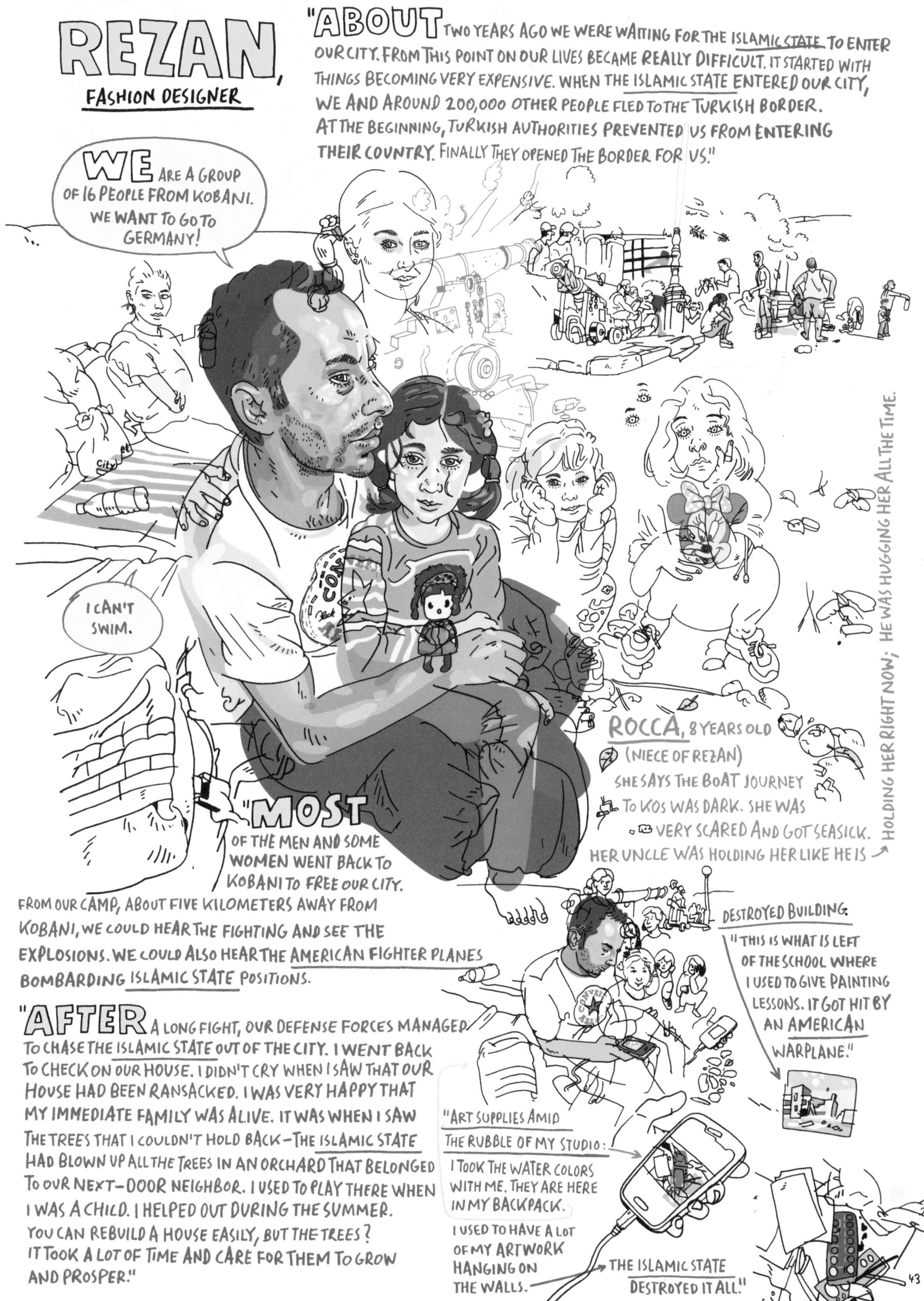
REZAN, FASHION DESIGNER
"ABOUT TWO YEARS AGO WE WERE WAITING FOR THE ISLAMIC STATE TO ENTER OUR CITY. FROM THIS POINT ON OUR LIVES BECAME REALLY DIFFICULT. IT STARTED WITH THINGS BECOMING VERY EXPENSIVE. WHEN THE ISLAMIC STATE ENTERED OUR CITY, WE AND AROUND 200,000 OTHER PEOPLE FLED TO THE TURKISH BORDER. AT THE BEGINNING, TURKISH AUTHORITIES PREVENTED US FROM ENTERING THEIR COUNTRY. FINALLY THEY OPENED THE BORDER FOR US."
WE ARE A GROUP OF 16 PEOPLE FROM KOBANI. WE WANT TO GO TO GERMANY!
I CAN'T SWIM.
ROCCA, 8 YEARS OLD (NIECE OF REZAN) SHE SAYS THE BOAT JOURNEY TO KOS WAS DARK. SHE WAS VERY SCARED AND GOT SEASICK. HER UNCLE WAS HOLDING HER LIKE HE IS → HOLDING HER RIGHT NOW; HE WAS HUGGING HER ALL THE TIME.
"MOST OF THE MEN AND SOME WOMEN WENT BACK TO KOBANI TO FREE OUR CITY. FROM OUR CAMP, ABOUT FIVE KILOMETERS AWAY FROM KOBANI, WE COULD HEAR THE FIGHTING AND SEE THE EXPLOSIONS. WE COULD ALSO HEAR THE AMERICAN FIGHTER PLANES BOMBARDING ISLAMIC STATE POSITIONS.
DESTROYED BUILDING: "THIS IS WHAT IS LEFT OF THE SCHOOL WHERE I USED TO GIVE PAINTING LESSONS. IT GOT HIT BY AN AMERICAN WARPLANE."
"AFTER A LONG FIGHT, OUR DEFENSE FORCES MANAGED TO CHASE THE ISLAMIC STATE OUT OF THE CITY. I WENT BACK TO CHECK ON OUR HOUSE. I DIDN'T CRY WHEN I SAW THAT OUR HOUSE HAD BEEN RANSACKED. I WAS VERY HAPPY THAT MY IMMEDIATE FAMILY WAS ALIVE. IT WAS WHEN I SAW THE TREES THAT I COULDN'T HOLD BACK—THE ISLAMIC STATE HAD BLOWN UP ALL THE TREES IN AN ORCHARD THAT BELONGED TO OUR NEXT-DOOR NEIGHBOR. I USED TO PLAY THERE WHEN I WAS A CHILD. I HELPED OUT DURING THE SUMMER. YOU CAN REBUILD A HOUSE EASILY, BUT THE TREES? IT TOOK A LOT OF TIME AND CARE FOR THEM TO GROW AND PROSPER."
"ART SUPPLIES AMID THE RUBBLE OF MY STUDIO: I TOOK THE WATER COLORS WITH ME. THEY ARE HERE IN MY BACKPACK.
I USED TO HAVE A LOT OF MY ARTWORK HANGING ON THE WALLS. → THE ISLAMIC STATE DESTROYED IT ALL."

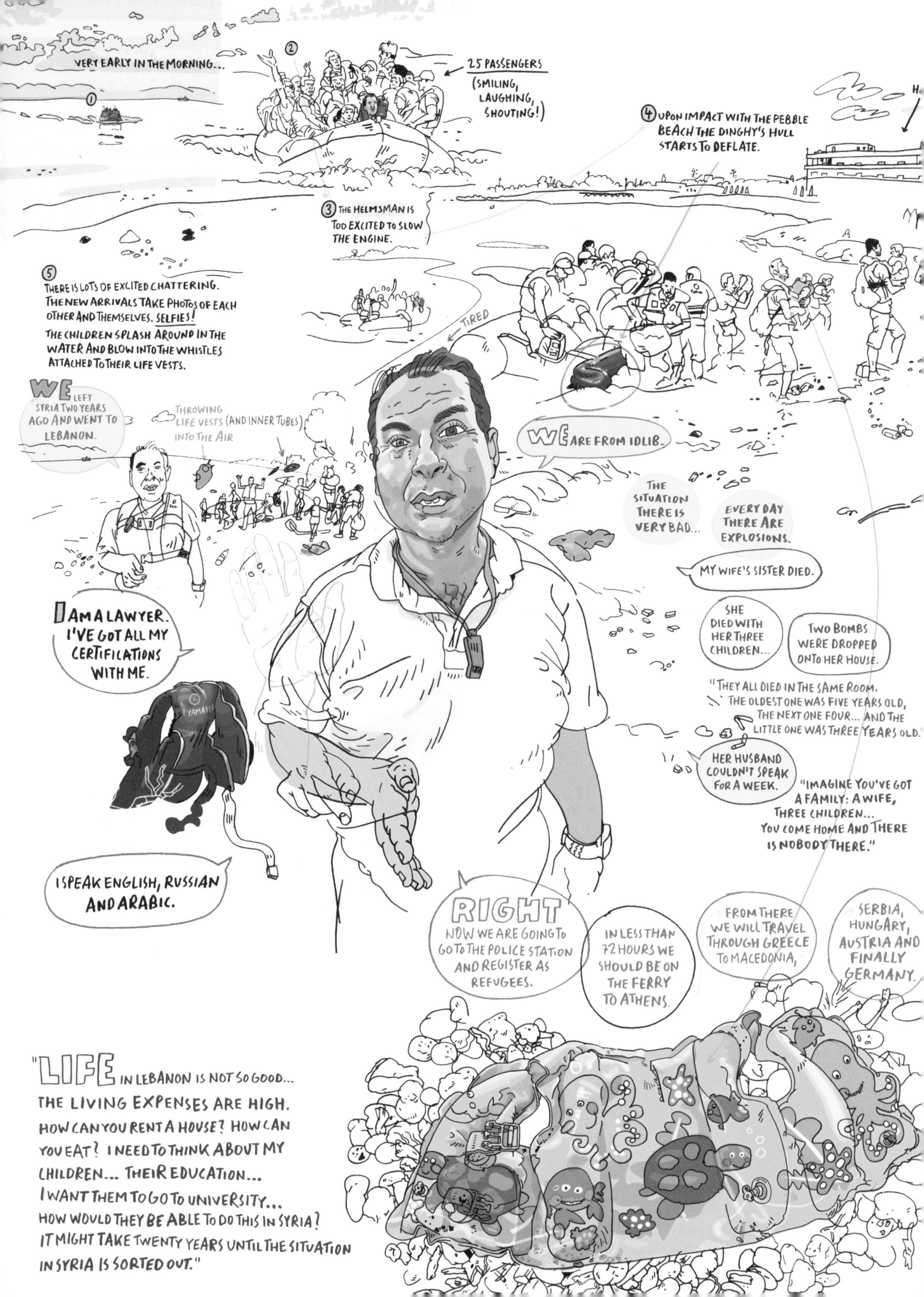
VERY EARLY IN THE MORNING...
①
②
25 PASSENGERS
(SMILING, LAUGHING, SHOUTING!)
③ THE HELMSMAN IS TOO EXCITED TO SLOW THE ENGINE.
④ UPON IMPACT WITH THE PEBBLE BEACH THE DINGHY'S HULL STARTS TO DEFLATE.
⑤ THERE IS LOTS OF EXCITED CHATTERING. THE NEW ARRIVALS TAKE PHOTOS OF EACH OTHER AND THEMSELVES. SELFIES! THE CHILDREN SPLASH AROUND IN THE WATER AND BLOW INTO THE WHISTLES ATTACHED TO THEIR LIFE VESTS.
TIRED
WE LEFT SYRIA TWO YEARS AGO AND WENT TO LEBANON.
THROWING LIFE VESTS (AND INNER TUBES) INTO THE AIR
WE ARE FROM IDLIB.
THE SITUATION THERE IS VERY BAD...
EVERY DAY THERE ARE EXPLOSIONS.
MY WIFE'S SISTER DIED.
I AM A LAWYER. I'VE GOT ALL MY CERTIFICATIONS WITH ME.
SHE DIED WITH HER THREE CHILDREN...
TWO BOMBS WERE DROPPED ONTO HER HOUSE.
"THEY ALL DIED IN THE SAME ROOM. THE OLDEST ONE WAS FIVE YEARS OLD, THE NEXT ONE FOUR... AND THE LITTLE ONE WAS THREE YEARS OLD.
YAMAHA
HER HUSBAND COULDN'T SPEAK FOR A WEEK.
"IMAGINE YOU'VE GOT A FAMILY: A WIFE, THREE CHILDREN... YOU COME HOME AND THERE IS NOBODY THERE."
I SPEAK ENGLISH, RUSSIAN AND ARABIC.
RIGHT NOW WE ARE GOING TO GO TO THE POLICE STATION AND REGISTER AS REFUGEES.
IN LESS THAN 72 HOURS WE SHOULD BE ON THE FERRY TO ATHENS.
FROM THERE WE WILL TRAVEL THROUGH GREECE TO MACEDONIA,
SERBIA, HUNGARY, AUSTRIA AND FINALLY GERMANY.
"LIFE IN LEBANON IS NOT SO GOOD... THE LIVING EXPENSES ARE HIGH. HOW CAN YOU RENT A HOUSE? HOW CAN YOU EAT? I NEED TO THINK ABOUT MY CHILDREN... THEIR EDUCATION... I WANT THEM TO GO TO UNIVERSITY... HOW WOULD THEY BE ABLE TO DO THIS IN SYRIA? IT MIGHT TAKE TWENTY YEARS UNTIL THE SITUATION IN SYRIA IS SORTED OUT."

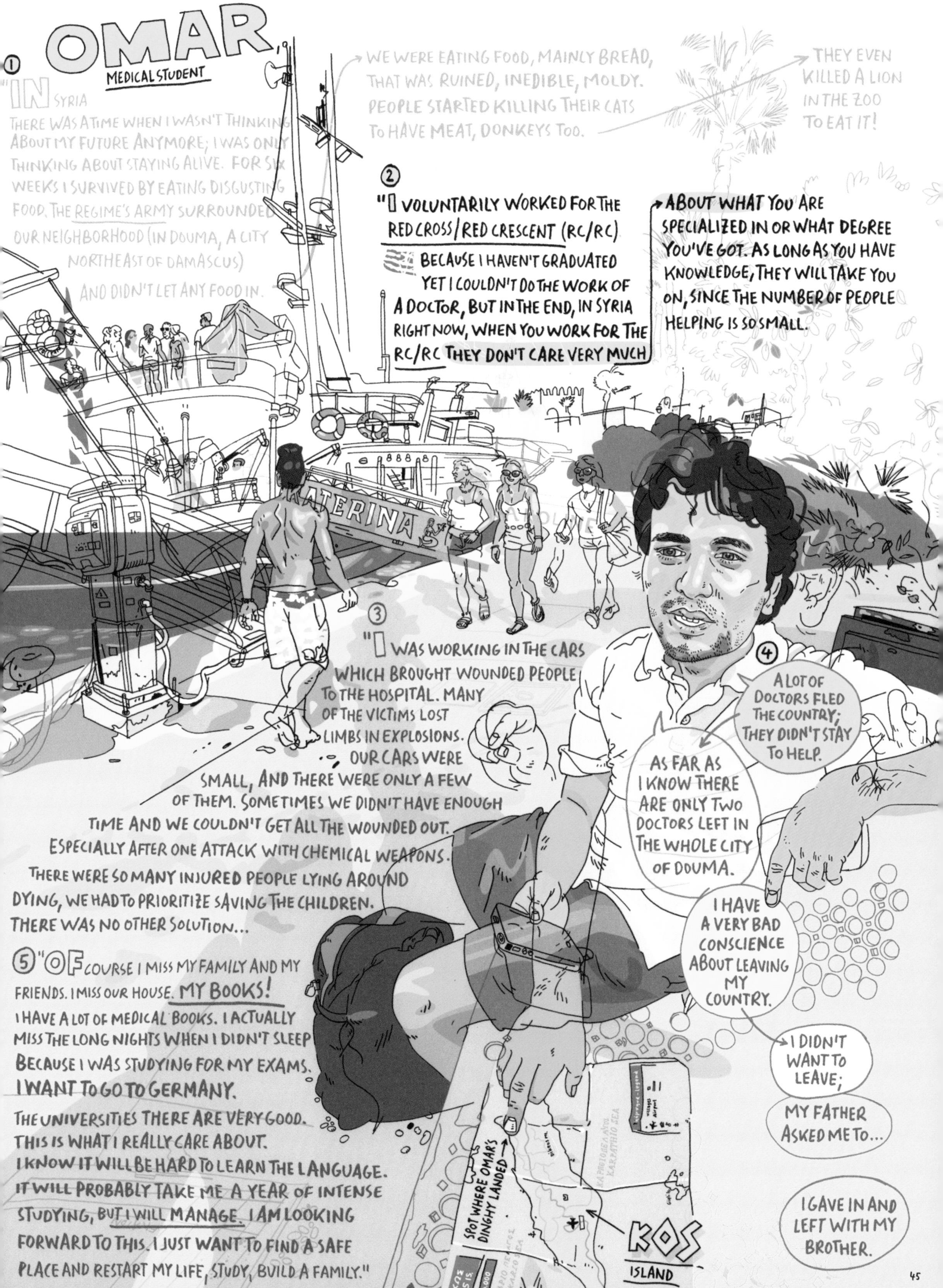

1
OMAR
MEDICAL STUDENT
"IN SYRIA
THERE WAS A TIME WHEN I WASN'T THINKING ABOUT MY FUTURE ANYMORE; I WAS ONLY THINKING ABOUT STAYING ALIVE. FOR SIX WEEKS I SURVIVED BY EATING DISGUSTING FOOD. THE REGIME'S ARMY SURROUNDED OUR NEIGHBORHOOD (IN DOUMA, A CITY NORTHEAST OF DAMASCUS)
AND DIDN'T LET ANY FOOD IN.
WE WERE EATING FOOD, MAINLY BREAD, THAT WAS RUINED, INEDIBLE, MOLDY. PEOPLE STARTED KILLING THEIR CATS TO HAVE MEAT, DONKEYS TOO.
THEY EVEN KILLED A LION IN THE ZOO TO EAT IT!
2
"I VOLUNTARILY WORKED FOR THE RED CROSS/RED CRESCENT (RC/RC)
BECAUSE I HAVEN'T GRADUATED YET I COULDN'T DO THE WORK OF A DOCTOR, BUT IN THE END, IN SYRIA RIGHT NOW, WHEN YOU WORK FOR THE RC/RC THEY DON'T CARE VERY MUCH
ABOUT WHAT YOU ARE SPECIALIZED IN OR WHAT DEGREE YOU'VE GOT. AS LONG AS YOU HAVE KNOWLEDGE, THEY WILL TAKE YOU ON, SINCE THE NUMBER OF PEOPLE HELPING IS SO SMALL.
ATERINA
3
"I WAS WORKING IN THE CARS WHICH BROUGHT WOUNDED PEOPLE TO THE HOSPITAL. MANY OF THE VICTIMS LOST LIMBS IN EXPLOSIONS. OUR CARS WERE SMALL, AND THERE WERE ONLY A FEW OF THEM. SOMETIMES WE DIDN'T HAVE ENOUGH TIME AND WE COULDN'T GET ALL THE WOUNDED OUT.
ESPECIALLY AFTER ONE ATTACK WITH CHEMICAL WEAPONS.
THERE WERE SO MANY INJURED PEOPLE LYING AROUND DYING, WE HAD TO PRIORITIZE SAVING THE CHILDREN. THERE WAS NO OTHER SOLUTION...
4
A LOT OF DOCTORS FLED THE COUNTRY; THEY DIDN'T STAY TO HELP.
AS FAR AS I KNOW THERE ARE ONLY TWO DOCTORS LEFT IN THE WHOLE CITY OF DOUMA.
I HAVE A VERY BAD CONSCIENCE ABOUT LEAVING MY COUNTRY.
I DIDN'T WANT TO LEAVE;
MY FATHER ASKED ME TO...
I GAVE IN AND LEFT WITH MY BROTHER.
5
"OF COURSE I MISS MY FAMILY AND MY FRIENDS. I MISS OUR HOUSE. MY BOOKS!
I HAVE A LOT OF MEDICAL BOOKS. I ACTUALLY MISS THE LONG NIGHTS WHEN I DIDN'T SLEEP BECAUSE I WAS STUDYING FOR MY EXAMS.
I WANT TO GO TO GERMANY.
THE UNIVERSITIES THERE ARE VERY GOOD. THIS IS WHAT I REALLY CARE ABOUT.
I KNOW IT WILL BE HARD TO LEARN THE LANGUAGE. IT WILL PROBABLY TAKE ME A YEAR OF INTENSE STUDYING, BUT I WILL MANAGE. I AM LOOKING FORWARD TO THIS. I JUST WANT TO FIND A SAFE PLACE AND RESTART MY LIFE, STUDY, BUILD A FAMILY."
SPOT WHERE OMAR'S DINGHY LANDED
KOS
ISLAND

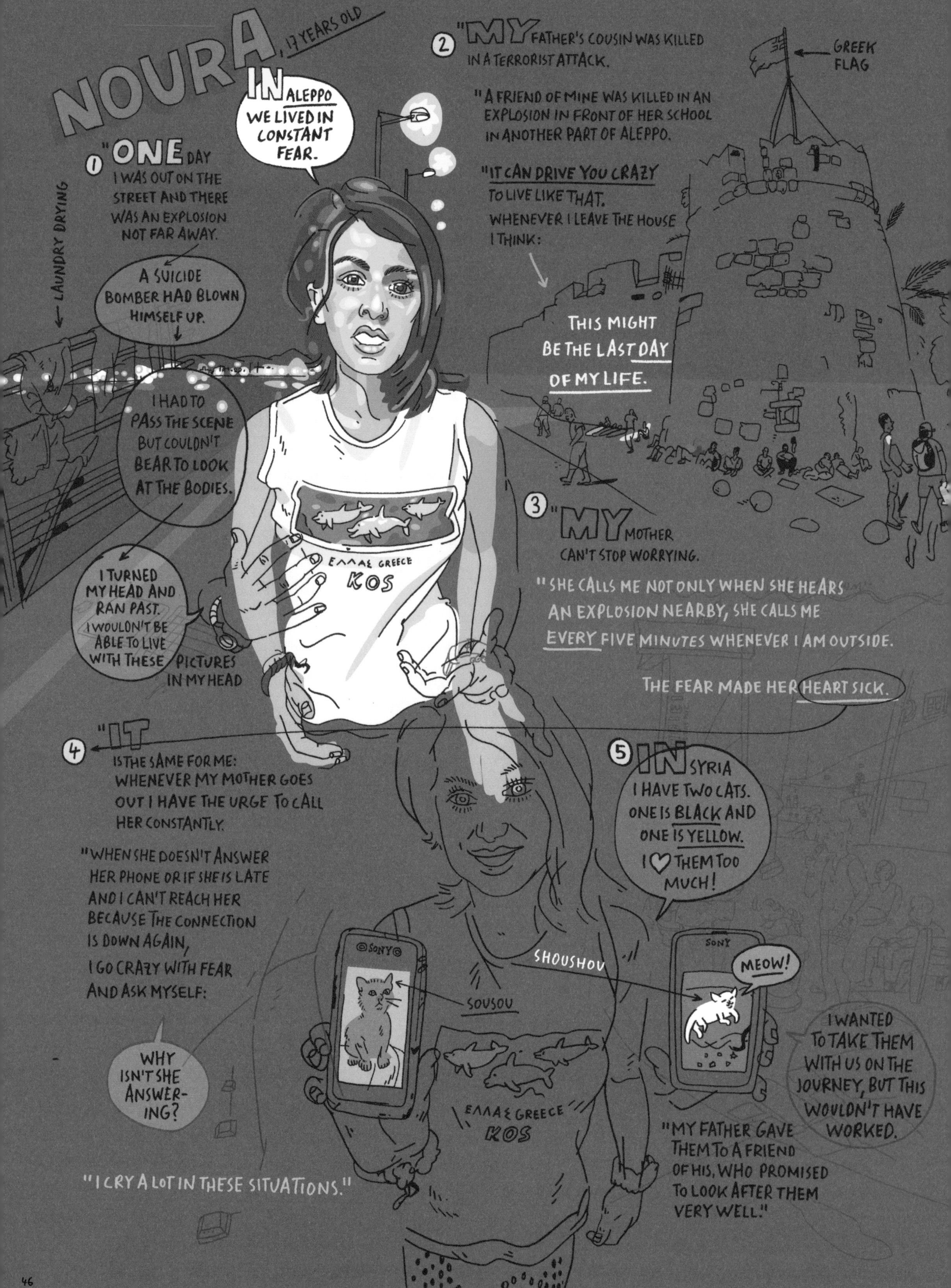
NOURA, 17 YEARS OLD
IN ALEPPO WE LIVED IN CONSTANT FEAR.
1 "ONE DAY I WAS OUT ON THE STREET AND THERE WAS AN EXPLOSION NOT FAR AWAY.
A SUICIDE BOMBER HAD BLOWN HIMSELF UP.
I HAD TO PASS THE SCENE BUT COULDN'T BEAR TO LOOK AT THE BODIES.
I TURNED MY HEAD AND RAN PAST. I WOULDN'T BE ABLE TO LIVE WITH THESE PICTURES IN MY HEAD
LAUNDRY DRYING
2 "MY FATHER'S COUSIN WAS KILLED IN A TERRORIST ATTACK.
"A FRIEND OF MINE WAS KILLED IN AN EXPLOSION IN FRONT OF HER SCHOOL IN ANOTHER PART OF ALEPPO.
"IT CAN DRIVE YOU CRAZY TO LIVE LIKE THAT. WHENEVER I LEAVE THE HOUSE I THINK:
THIS MIGHT BE THE LAST DAY OF MY LIFE.
GREEK FLAG
ΕΛΛΑΣ GREECE KOS
3 "MY MOTHER CAN'T STOP WORRYING.
"SHE CALLS ME NOT ONLY WHEN SHE HEARS AN EXPLOSION NEARBY, SHE CALLS ME EVERY FIVE MINUTES WHENEVER I AM OUTSIDE.
THE FEAR MADE HER HEART SICK.
4 "IT IS THE SAME FOR ME: WHENEVER MY MOTHER GOES OUT I HAVE THE URGE TO CALL HER CONSTANTLY.
"WHEN SHE DOESN'T ANSWER HER PHONE OR IF SHE IS LATE AND I CAN'T REACH HER BECAUSE THE CONNECTION IS DOWN AGAIN, I GO CRAZY WITH FEAR AND ASK MYSELF:
WHY ISN'T SHE ANSWER-ING?
"I CRY A LOT IN THESE SITUATIONS."
5 "IN SYRIA I HAVE TWO CATS. ONE IS BLACK AND ONE IS YELLOW. I ♥ THEM TOO MUCH!
SONY
SOUSOU
SHOUSHOU
SONY
MEOW!
ΕΛΛΑΣ GREECE KOS
I WANTED TO TAKE THEM WITH US ON THE JOURNEY, BUT THIS WOULDN'T HAVE WORKED.
"MY FATHER GAVE THEM TO A FRIEND OF HIS, WHO PROMISED TO LOOK AFTER THEM VERY WELL."

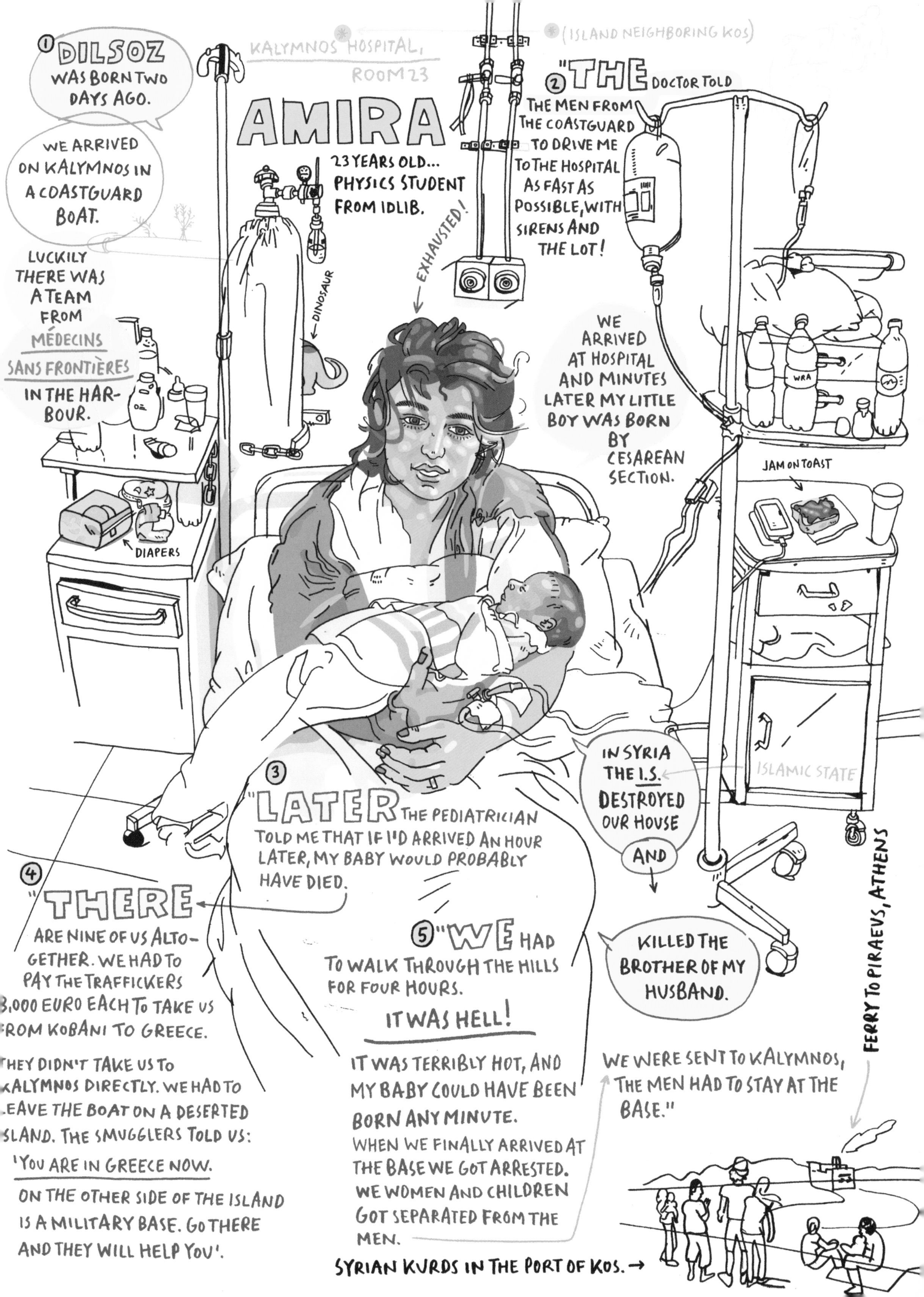

(ISLAND NEIGHBORING KOS)
KALYMNOS HOSPITAL, ROOM 23
AMIRA
23 YEARS OLD... PHYSICS STUDENT FROM IDLIB.
EXHAUSTED!
DINOSAUR
① DILSOZ WAS BORN TWO DAYS AGO.
WE ARRIVED ON KALYMNOS IN A COASTGUARD BOAT.
LUCKILY THERE WAS A TEAM FROM MÉDECINS SANS FRONTIÈRES IN THE HARBOUR.
② "THE DOCTOR TOLD THE MEN FROM THE COASTGUARD TO DRIVE ME TO THE HOSPITAL AS FAST AS POSSIBLE, WITH SIRENS AND THE LOT!
WE ARRIVED AT HOSPITAL AND MINUTES LATER MY LITTLE BOY WAS BORN BY CESAREAN SECTION.
WRA
JAM ON TOAST
DIAPERS
IN SYRIA THE I.S. DESTROYED OUR HOUSE
ISLAMIC STATE
AND
KILLED THE BROTHER OF MY HUSBAND.
③ "LATER THE PEDIATRICIAN TOLD ME THAT IF I'D ARRIVED AN HOUR LATER, MY BABY WOULD PROBABLY HAVE DIED.
④ "THERE ARE NINE OF US ALTOGETHER. WE HAD TO PAY THE TRAFFICKERS 3,000 EURO EACH TO TAKE US ROM KOBANI TO GREECE.
HEY DIDN'T TAKE US TO ALYMNOS DIRECTLY. WE HAD TO EAVE THE BOAT ON A DESERTED SLAND. THE SMUGGLERS TOLD US:
'YOU ARE IN GREECE NOW.
ON THE OTHER SIDE OF THE ISLAND IS A MILITARY BASE. GO THERE AND THEY WILL HELP YOU'.
⑤ "WE HAD TO WALK THROUGH THE HILLS FOR FOUR HOURS.
IT WAS HELL!
IT WAS TERRIBLY HOT, AND MY BABY COULD HAVE BEEN BORN ANY MINUTE.
WHEN WE FINALLY ARRIVED AT THE BASE WE GOT ARRESTED. WE WOMEN AND CHILDREN GOT SEPARATED FROM THE MEN.
WE WERE SENT TO KALYMNOS, THE MEN HAD TO STAY AT THE BASE."
FERRY TO PIRAEUS, ATHENS
SYRIAN KURDS IN THE PORT OF KOS. →

FRANCE

P&O

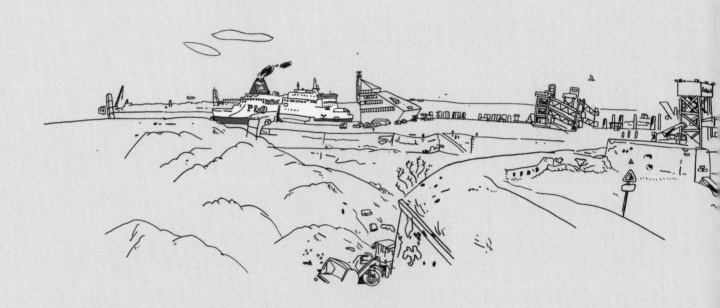

THE CALAIS 'JUNGLE CAMP', FRANCE

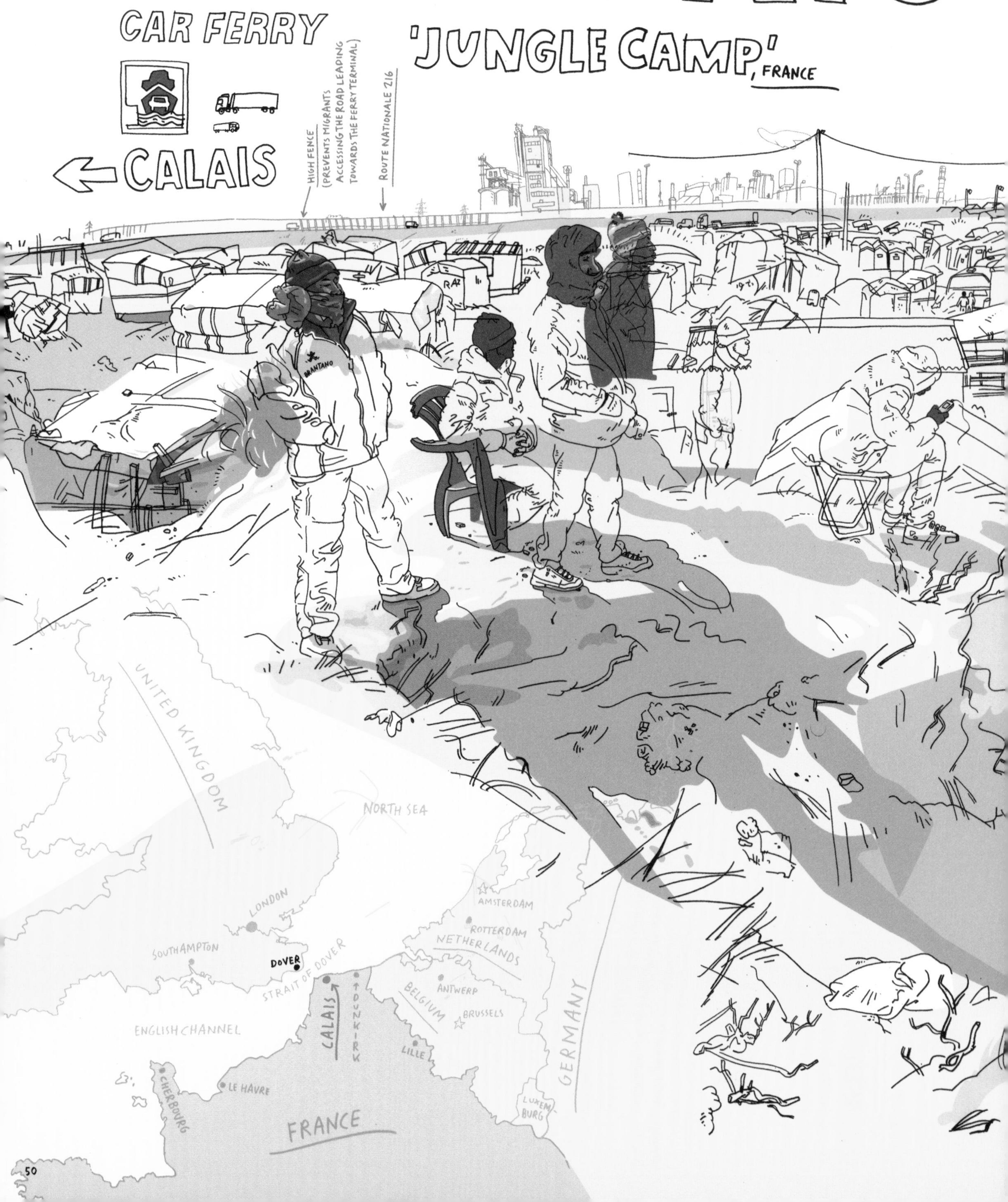

CAR FERRY
CALAIS
HIGH FENCE (PREVENTS MIGRANTS ACCESSING THE ROAD LEADING TOWARDS THE FERRY TERMINAL)
ROUTE NATIONALE 216
BRANTANO
UNITED KINGDOM
NORTH SEA
LONDON
AMSTERDAM
ROTTERDAM
NETHERLANDS
SOUTHAMPTON
DOVER
STRAIT OF DOVER
CALAIS
DUNKIRK
BELGIUM
ANTWERP
BRUSSELS
GERMANY
ENGLISH CHANNEL
LILLE
CHERBOURG
LE HAVRE
LUXEMBURG
FRANCE

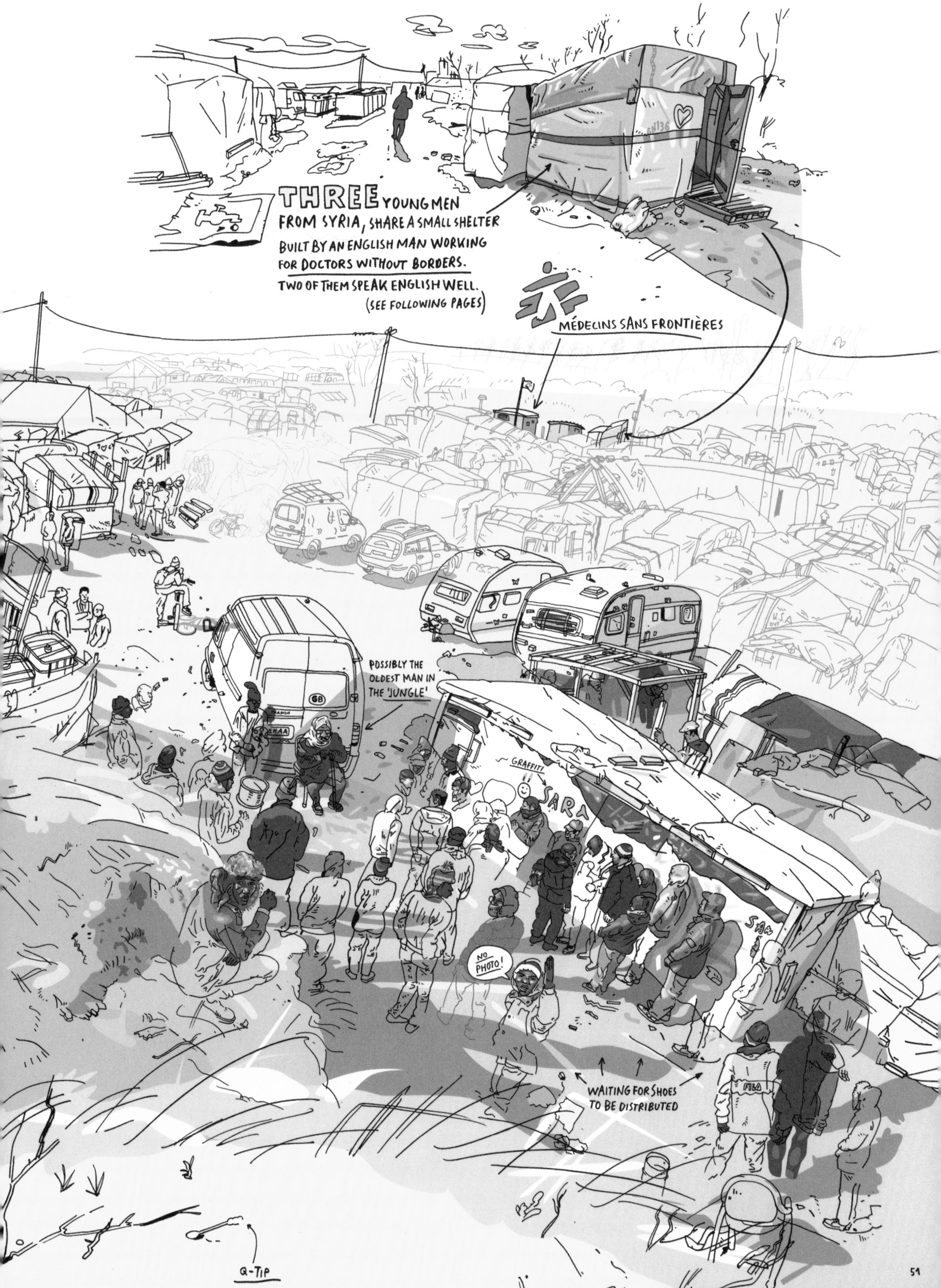
THREE YOUNG MEN FROM SYRIA, SHARE A SMALL SHELTER BUILT BY AN ENGLISH MAN WORKING FOR DOCTORS WITHOUT BORDERS.
TWO OF THEM SPEAK ENGLISH WELL.
(SEE FOLLOWING PAGES)
MÉDECINS SANS FRONTIÈRES
POSSIBLY THE OLDEST MAN IN THE 'JUNGLE'
GRAFFITI
SARA
NO PHOTO!
WAITING FOR SHOES TO BE DISTRIBUTED
Q-TIP

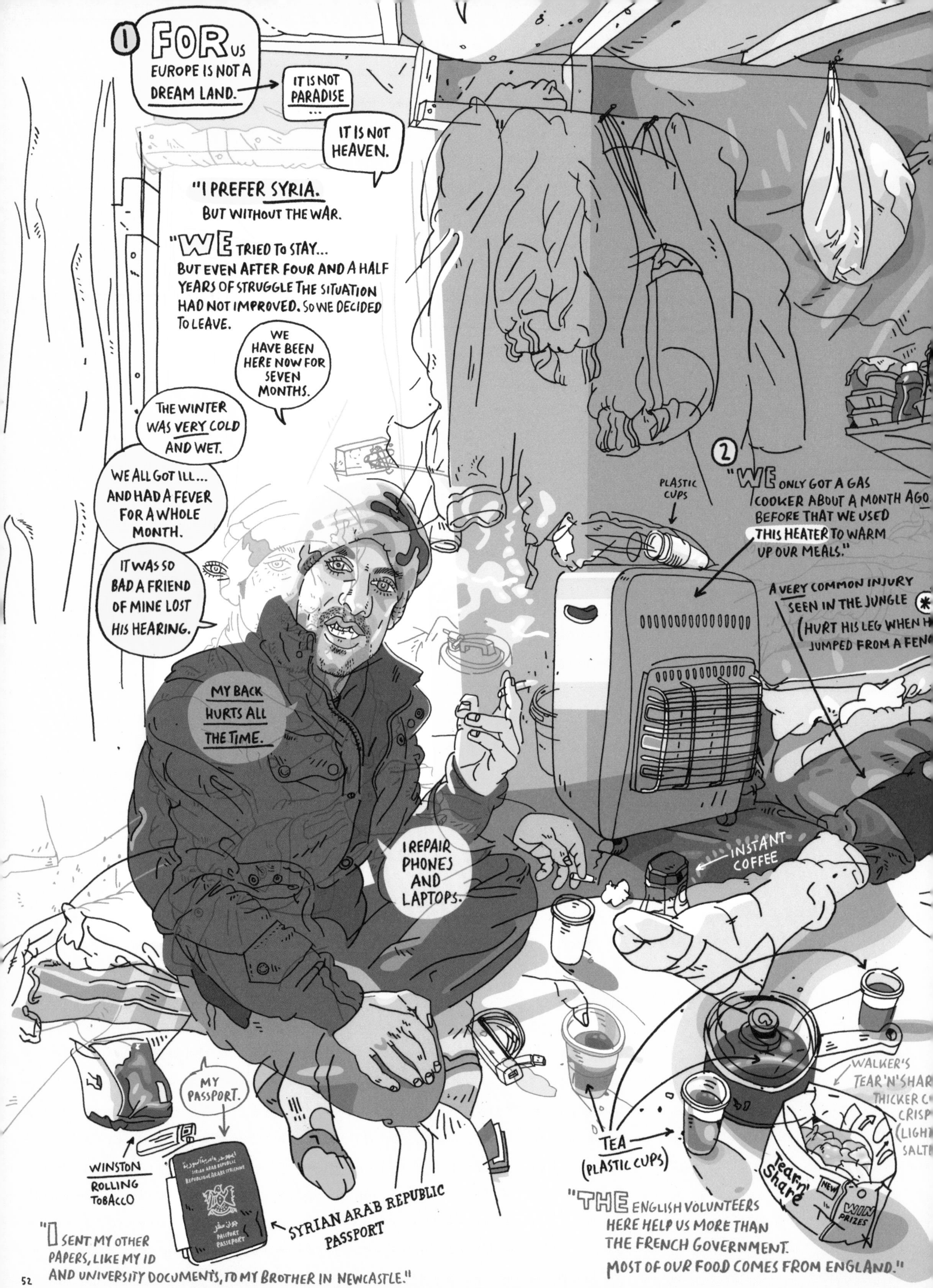

1 FOR US EUROPE IS NOT A DREAM LAND.
IT IS NOT PARADISE ...
IT IS NOT HEAVEN.
"I PREFER SYRIA. BUT WITHOUT THE WAR.
"WE TRIED TO STAY... BUT EVEN AFTER FOUR AND A HALF YEARS OF STRUGGLE THE SITUATION HAD NOT IMPROVED. SO WE DECIDED TO LEAVE.
WE HAVE BEEN HERE NOW FOR SEVEN MONTHS.
THE WINTER WAS VERY COLD AND WET.
WE ALL GOT ILL... AND HAD A FEVER FOR A WHOLE MONTH.
IT WAS SO BAD A FRIEND OF MINE LOST HIS HEARING.
MY BACK HURTS ALL THE TIME.
I REPAIR PHONES AND LAPTOPS.
2 "WE ONLY GOT A GAS COOKER ABOUT A MONTH AGO. BEFORE THAT WE USED THIS HEATER TO WARM UP OUR MEALS."
PLASTIC CUPS
A VERY COMMON INJURY SEEN IN THE JUNGLE
INSTANT COFFEE
MY PASSPORT.
WINSTON ROLLING TOBACCO
SYRIAN ARAB REPUBLIC PASSPORT
TEA (PLASTIC CUPS)
"I SENT MY OTHER PAPERS, LIKE MY ID AND UNIVERSITY DOCUMENTS, TO MY BROTHER IN NEWCASTLE."
"THE ENGLISH VOLUNTEERS HERE HELP US MORE THAN THE FRENCH GOVERNMENT. MOST OF OUR FOOD COMES FROM ENGLAND."
Tear 'n' Share
NEW
WIN PRIZES

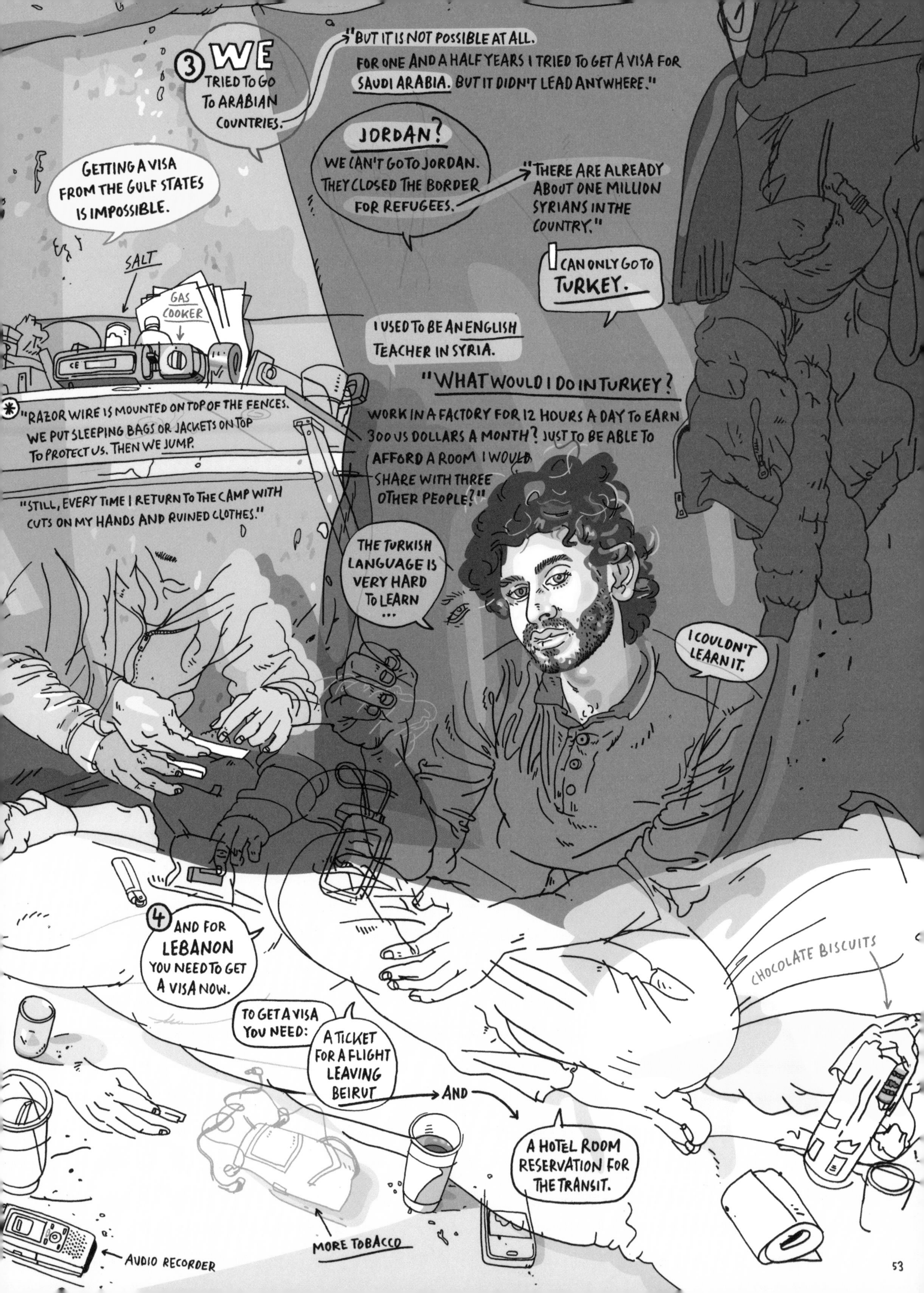

③ WE TRIED TO GO TO ARABIAN COUNTRIES.
"BUT IT IS NOT POSSIBLE AT ALL. FOR ONE AND A HALF YEARS I TRIED TO GET A VISA FOR SAUDI ARABIA. BUT IT DIDN'T LEAD ANYWHERE."
GETTING A VISA FROM THE GULF STATES IS IMPOSSIBLE.
JORDAN? WE CAN'T GO TO JORDAN. THEY CLOSED THE BORDER FOR REFUGEES.
"THERE ARE ALREADY ABOUT ONE MILLION SYRIANS IN THE COUNTRY."
I CAN ONLY GO TO TURKEY.
SALT
GAS COOKER
I USED TO BE AN ENGLISH TEACHER IN SYRIA.
"WHAT WOULD I DO IN TURKEY?
WORK IN A FACTORY FOR 12 HOURS A DAY TO EARN 300 US DOLLARS A MONTH? JUST TO BE ABLE TO AFFORD A ROOM I WOULD SHARE WITH THREE OTHER PEOPLE?"
* "RAZOR WIRE IS MOUNTED ON TOP OF THE FENCES. WE PUT SLEEPING BAGS OR JACKETS ON TOP TO PROTECT US. THEN WE JUMP.
"STILL, EVERY TIME I RETURN TO THE CAMP WITH CUTS ON MY HANDS AND RUINED CLOTHES."
THE TURKISH LANGUAGE IS VERY HARD TO LEARN ...
I COULDN'T LEARN IT.
④ AND FOR LEBANON YOU NEED TO GET A VISA NOW.
TO GET A VISA YOU NEED:
A TICKET FOR A FLIGHT LEAVING BEIRUT
AND
A HOTEL ROOM RESERVATION FOR THE TRANSIT.
CHOCOLATE BISCUITS
MORE TOBACCO
AUDIO RECORDER

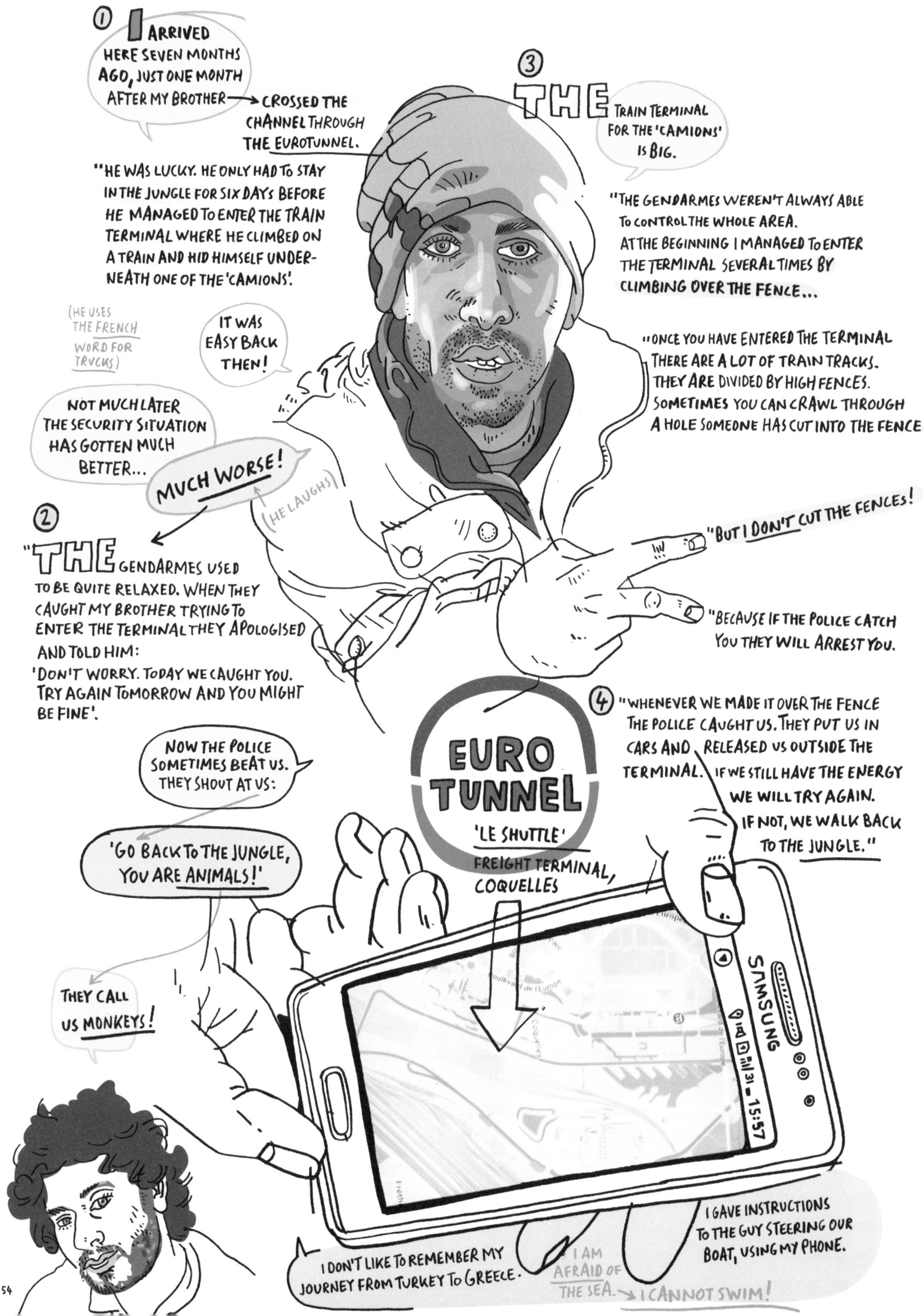

① I ARRIVED HERE SEVEN MONTHS AGO, JUST ONE MONTH AFTER MY BROTHER
CROSSED THE CHANNEL THROUGH THE EUROTUNNEL.
"HE WAS LUCKY. HE ONLY HAD TO STAY IN THE JUNGLE FOR SIX DAYS BEFORE HE MANAGED TO ENTER THE TRAIN TERMINAL WHERE HE CLIMBED ON A TRAIN AND HID HIMSELF UNDERNEATH ONE OF THE 'CAMIONS'.
(HE USES THE FRENCH WORD FOR TRUCKS)
IT WAS EASY BACK THEN!
NOT MUCH LATER THE SECURITY SITUATION HAS GOTTEN MUCH BETTER...
MUCH WORSE!
(HE LAUGHS)
② "THE GENDARMES USED TO BE QUITE RELAXED. WHEN THEY CAUGHT MY BROTHER TRYING TO ENTER THE TERMINAL THEY APOLOGISED AND TOLD HIM:
'DON'T WORRY. TODAY WE CAUGHT YOU. TRY AGAIN TOMORROW AND YOU MIGHT BE FINE'.
③ THE TRAIN TERMINAL FOR THE 'CAMIONS' IS BIG.
"THE GENDARMES WEREN'T ALWAYS ABLE TO CONTROL THE WHOLE AREA. AT THE BEGINNING I MANAGED TO ENTER THE TERMINAL SEVERAL TIMES BY CLIMBING OVER THE FENCE...
"ONCE YOU HAVE ENTERED THE TERMINAL THERE ARE A LOT OF TRAIN TRACKS. THEY ARE DIVIDED BY HIGH FENCES. SOMETIMES YOU CAN CRAWL THROUGH A HOLE SOMEONE HAS CUT INTO THE FENCE...
"BUT I DON'T CUT THE FENCES!
"BECAUSE IF THE POLICE CATCH YOU THEY WILL ARREST YOU.
④ "WHENEVER WE MADE IT OVER THE FENCE THE POLICE CAUGHT US. THEY PUT US IN CARS AND RELEASED US OUTSIDE THE TERMINAL. IF WE STILL HAVE THE ENERGY WE WILL TRY AGAIN. IF NOT, WE WALK BACK TO THE JUNGLE."
EURO TUNNEL
'LE SHUTTLE'
FREIGHT TERMINAL, COQUELLES
NOW THE POLICE SOMETIMES BEAT US. THEY SHOUT AT US:
'GO BACK TO THE JUNGLE, YOU ARE ANIMALS!'
THEY CALL US MONKEYS!
SAMSUNG
15:57
I GAVE INSTRUCTIONS TO THE GUY STEERING OUR BOAT, USING MY PHONE.
I DON'T LIKE TO REMEMBER MY JOURNEY FROM TURKEY TO GREECE.
I AM AFRAID OF THE SEA.
I CANNOT SWIM!

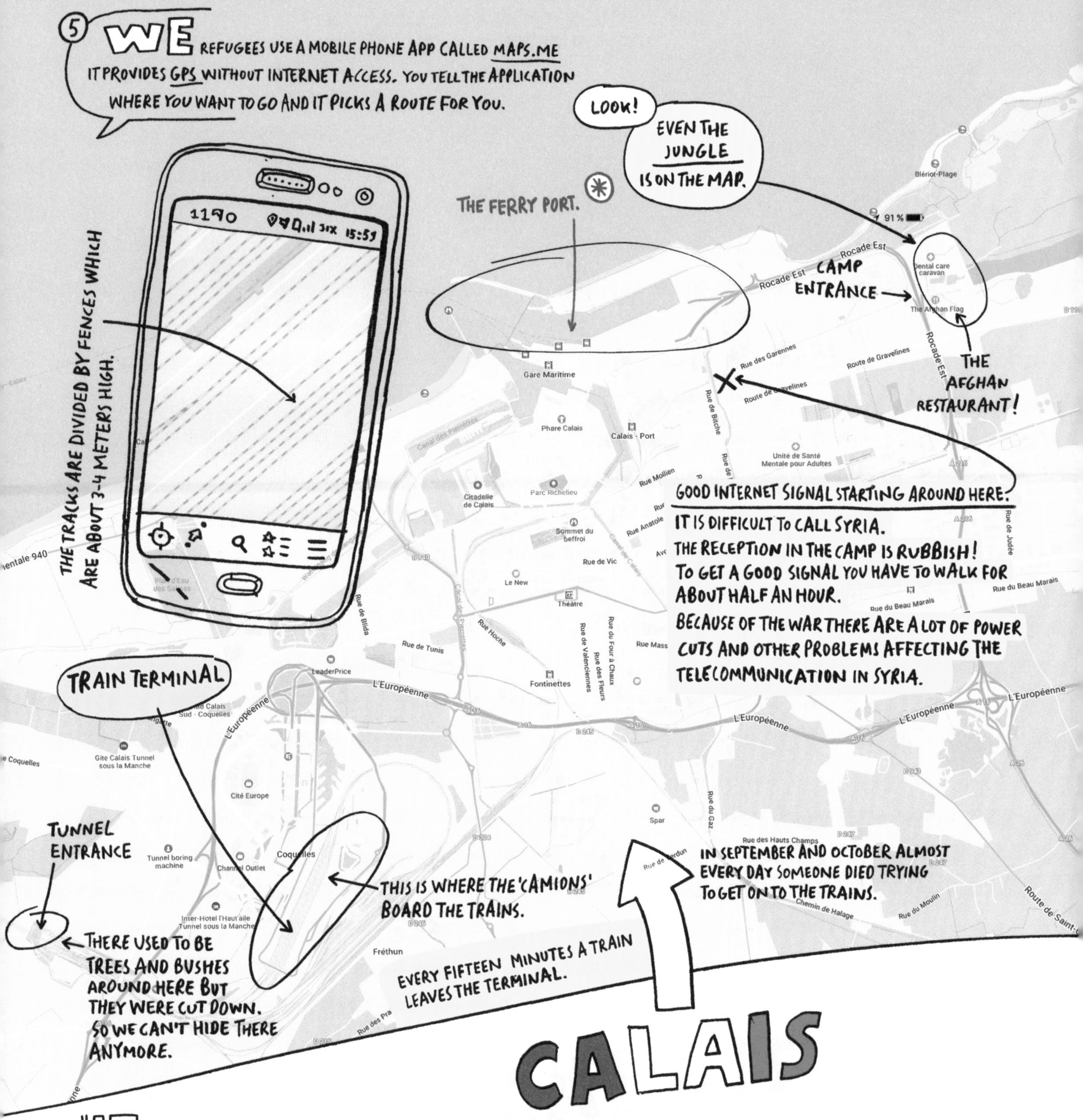

5 WE REFUGEES USE A MOBILE PHONE APP CALLED MAPS.ME IT PROVIDES GPS WITHOUT INTERNET ACCESS. YOU TELL THE APPLICATION WHERE YOU WANT TO GO AND IT PICKS A ROUTE FOR YOU.
LOOK!
EVEN THE JUNGLE IS ON THE MAP.
THE FERRY PORT.
CAMP ENTRANCE
THE AFGHAN RESTAURANT!
THE TRACKS ARE DIVIDED BY FENCES WHICH ARE ABOUT 3-4 METERS HIGH.
GOOD INTERNET SIGNAL STARTING AROUND HERE.
IT IS DIFFICULT TO CALL SYRIA. THE RECEPTION IN THE CAMP IS RUBBISH! TO GET A GOOD SIGNAL YOU HAVE TO WALK FOR ABOUT HALF AN HOUR. BECAUSE OF THE WAR THERE ARE A LOT OF POWER CUTS AND OTHER PROBLEMS AFFECTING THE TELECOMMUNICATION IN SYRIA.
TRAIN TERMINAL
TUNNEL ENTRANCE
THERE USED TO BE TREES AND BUSHES AROUND HERE BUT THEY WERE CUT DOWN. SO WE CAN'T HIDE THERE ANYMORE.
THIS IS WHERE THE 'CAMIONS' BOARD THE TRAINS.
EVERY FIFTEEN MINUTES A TRAIN LEAVES THE TERMINAL.
IN SEPTEMBER AND OCTOBER ALMOST EVERY DAY SOMEONE DIED TRYING TO GET ONTO THE TRAINS.
CALAIS

6 "IT IS A THREE TO FOUR HOUR WALK FROM THE 'JUNGLE' THROUGH THE TOWN TO THE TERMINAL. WHEN WE ARRIVE THERE WE ARE TIRED AND IT IS EASY FOR THE POLICE TO CATCH US. WE USED TO DO THIS EVERY NIGHT UNTIL ABOUT A MONTH AGO.

"NOW THERE ARE MORE THAN A 1,000 GENDARMES... EVEN THE ARMY IS GUARDING THE TERMINAL! WHEN I ARRIVED IN THE 'JUNGLE', AROUND 50 PEOPLE MADE THE CROSSING THROUGH THE TUNNEL EVERY NIGHT. NOW IT IS MAYBE ONE PERSON EVERY THREE DAYS."

* "TRYING TO HIDE ON A TRUCK AND GOING THROUGH THE PORT IS DIFFICULT... THERE ARE THREE SCANNERS. TWO RUN BY THE FRENCH POLICE AND ONE BY THE UK BORDER FORCE. IT IS DIFFICULT TO PASS THEM. YOU CAN SPEND TEN HOURS HIDDEN ON A TRUCK UNTIL THE POLICE CATCH YOU AND SEND YOU BACK TO THE 'JUNGLE'."

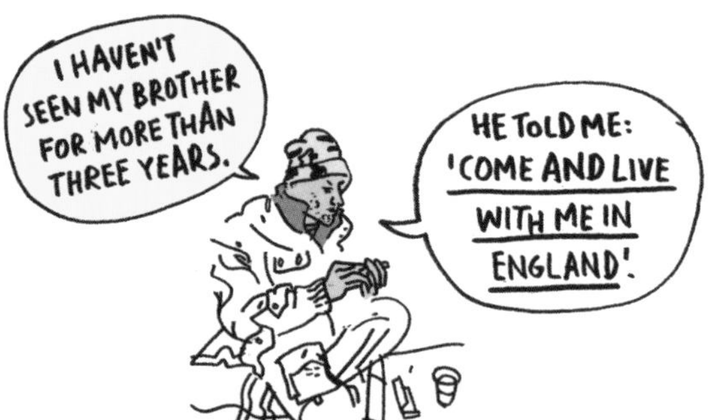

I HAVEN'T SEEN MY BROTHER FOR MORE THAN THREE YEARS.
HE TOLD ME: 'COME AND LIVE WITH ME IN ENGLAND'.

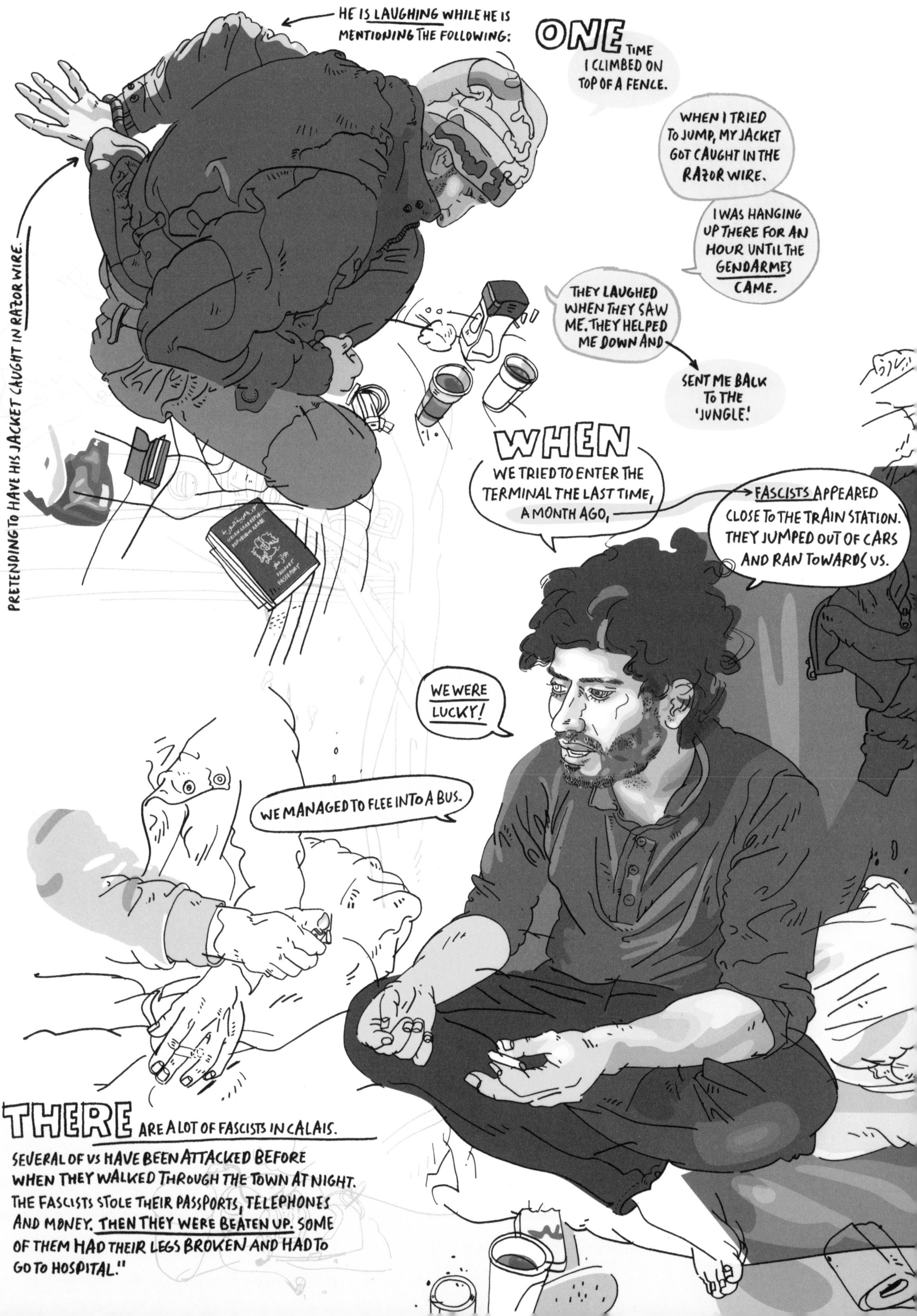
HE IS LAUGHING WHILE HE IS MENTIONING THE FOLLOWING:
PRETENDING TO HAVE HIS JACKET CAUGHT IN RAZOR WIRE.
ONE TIME I CLIMBED ON TOP OF A FENCE.
WHEN I TRIED TO JUMP, MY JACKET GOT CAUGHT IN THE RAZOR WIRE.
I WAS HANGING UP THERE FOR AN HOUR UNTIL THE GENDARMES CAME.
THEY LAUGHED WHEN THEY SAW ME. THEY HELPED ME DOWN AND
SENT ME BACK TO THE 'JUNGLE.'
SYRIAN ARAB REPUBLIC
PASSPORT
WHEN WE TRIED TO ENTER THE TERMINAL THE LAST TIME, A MONTH AGO,
FASCISTS APPEARED CLOSE TO THE TRAIN STATION. THEY JUMPED OUT OF CARS AND RAN TOWARDS US.
WE WERE LUCKY!
WE MANAGED TO FLEE INTO A BUS.
"THERE ARE A LOT OF FASCISTS IN CALAIS.
SEVERAL OF US HAVE BEEN ATTACKED BEFORE WHEN THEY WALKED THROUGH THE TOWN AT NIGHT. THE FASCISTS STOLE THEIR PASSPORTS, TELEPHONES AND MONEY. THEN THEY WERE BEATEN UP. SOME OF THEM HAD THEIR LEGS BROKEN AND HAD TO GO TO HOSPITAL."

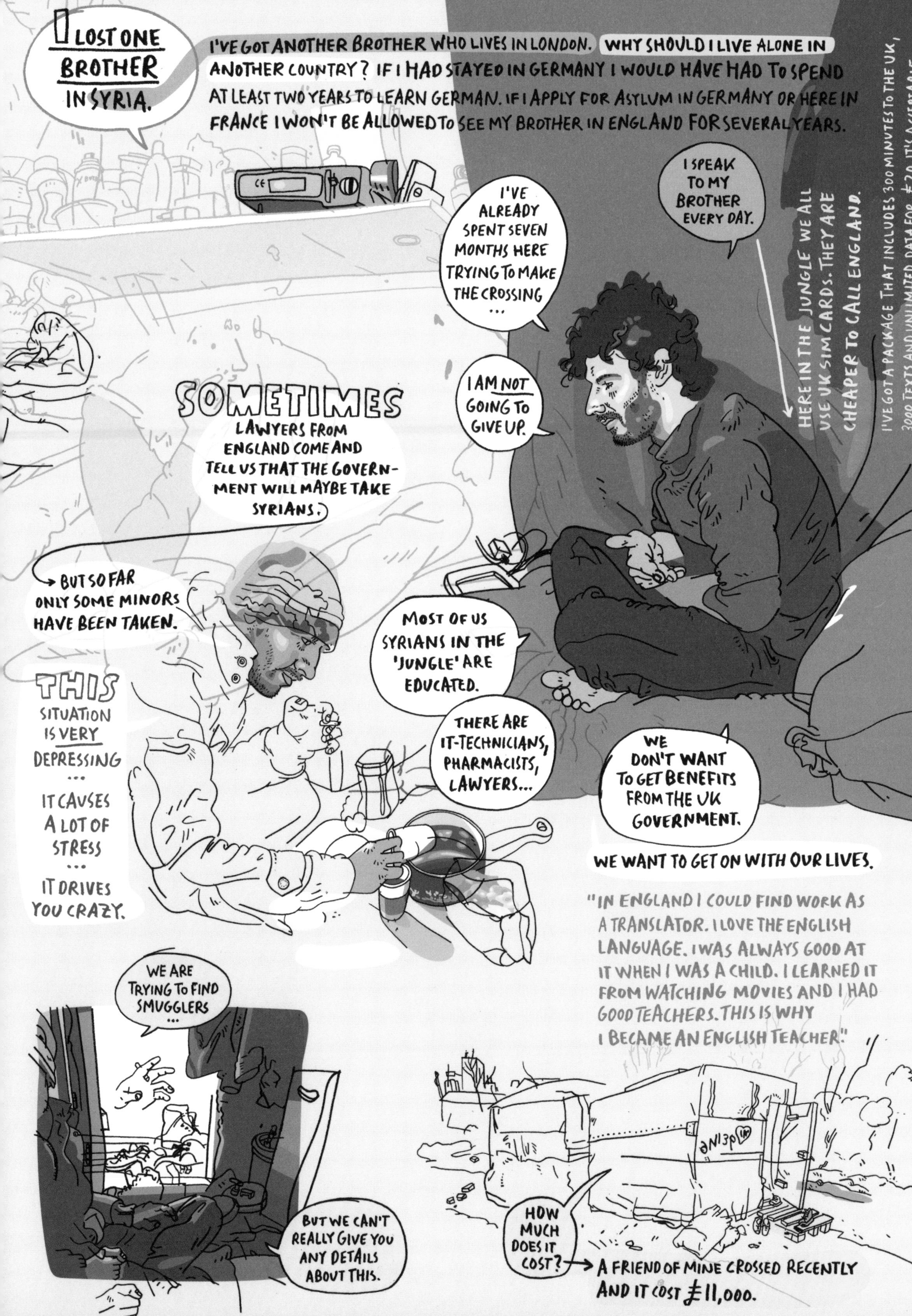
I LOST ONE BROTHER IN SYRIA.
I'VE GOT ANOTHER BROTHER WHO LIVES IN LONDON. WHY SHOULD I LIVE ALONE IN ANOTHER COUNTRY? IF I HAD STAYED IN GERMANY I WOULD HAVE HAD TO SPEND AT LEAST TWO YEARS TO LEARN GERMAN. IF I APPLY FOR ASYLUM IN GERMANY OR HERE IN FRANCE I WON'T BE ALLOWED TO SEE MY BROTHER IN ENGLAND FOR SEVERAL YEARS.
I'VE ALREADY SPENT SEVEN MONTHS HERE TRYING TO MAKE THE CROSSING…
I SPEAK TO MY BROTHER EVERY DAY.
HERE IN THE JUNGLE WE ALL USE UK SIM CARDS. THEY ARE CHEAPER TO CALL ENGLAND.
I'VE GOT A PACKAGE THAT INCLUDES 300 MINUTES TO THE UK, 3000 TEXTS AND UNLIMITED DATA FOR £20. IT'S ACCEPTABLE.
I AM NOT GOING TO GIVE UP.
SOMETIMES LAWYERS FROM ENGLAND COME AND TELL US THAT THE GOVERNMENT WILL MAYBE TAKE SYRIANS.
BUT SO FAR ONLY SOME MINORS HAVE BEEN TAKEN.
MOST OF US SYRIANS IN THE 'JUNGLE' ARE EDUCATED.
THERE ARE IT-TECHNICIANS, PHARMACISTS, LAWYERS…
WE DON'T WANT TO GET BENEFITS FROM THE UK GOVERNMENT.
WE WANT TO GET ON WITH OUR LIVES.
THIS SITUATION IS VERY DEPRESSING… IT CAUSES A LOT OF STRESS… IT DRIVES YOU CRAZY.
"IN ENGLAND I COULD FIND WORK AS A TRANSLATOR. I LOVE THE ENGLISH LANGUAGE. I WAS ALWAYS GOOD AT IT WHEN I WAS A CHILD. I LEARNED IT FROM WATCHING MOVIES AND I HAD GOOD TEACHERS. THIS IS WHY I BECAME AN ENGLISH TEACHER."
WE ARE TRYING TO FIND SMUGGLERS…
BUT WE CAN'T REALLY GIVE YOU ANY DETAILS ABOUT THIS.
HOW MUCH DOES IT COST?
A FRIEND OF MINE CROSSED RECENTLY AND IT COST £11,000.

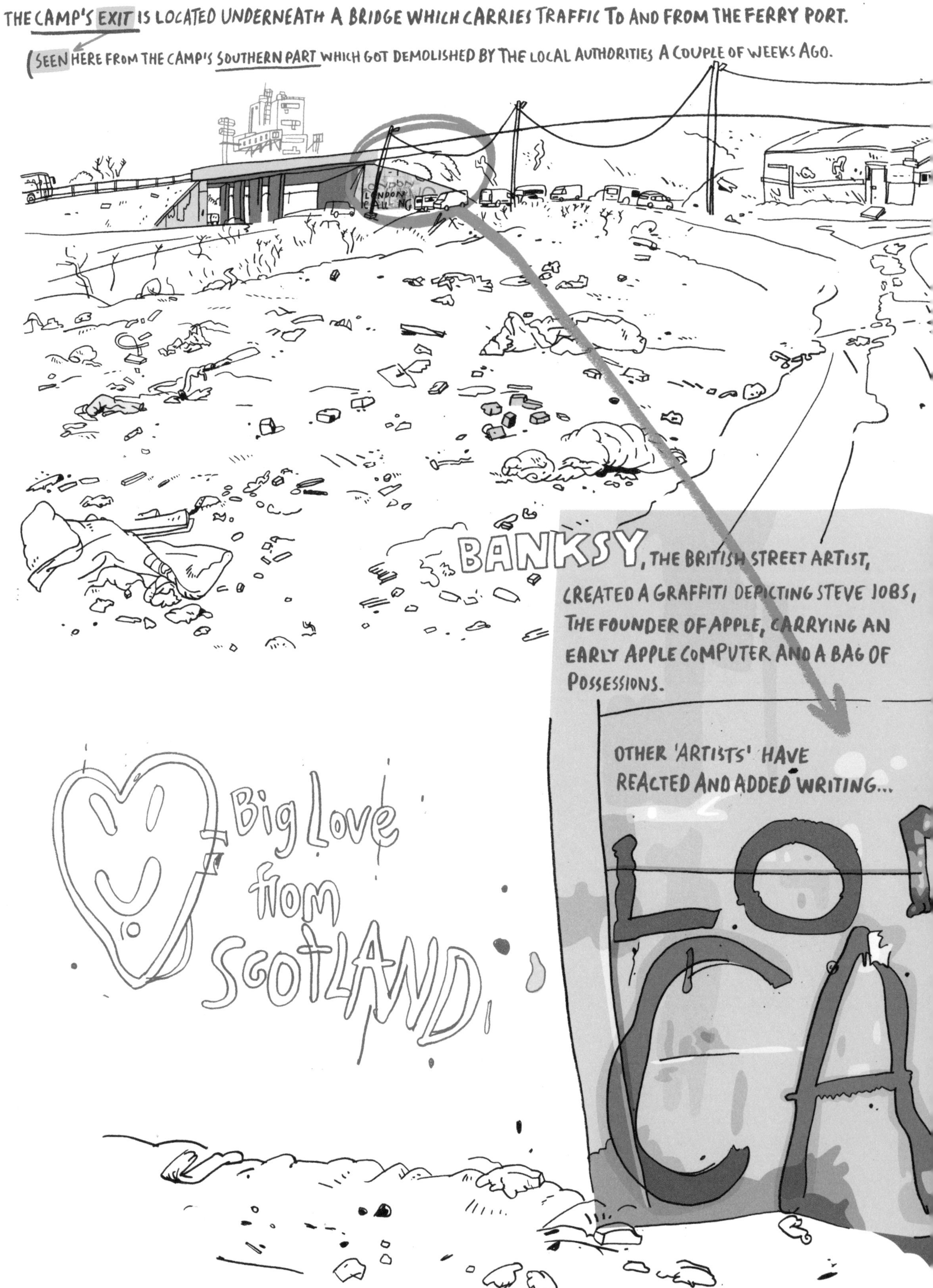
THE CAMP'S EXIT IS LOCATED UNDERNEATH A BRIDGE WHICH CARRIES TRAFFIC TO AND FROM THE FERRY PORT.
(SEEN HERE FROM THE CAMP'S SOUTHERN PART WHICH GOT DEMOLISHED BY THE LOCAL AUTHORITIES A COUPLE OF WEEKS AGO.
BANKSY, THE BRITISH STREET ARTIST, CREATED A GRAFFITI DEPICTING STEVE JOBS, THE FOUNDER OF APPLE, CARRYING AN EARLY APPLE COMPUTER AND A BAG OF POSSESSIONS.
OTHER 'ARTISTS' HAVE REACTED AND ADDED WRITING...
Big Love from SCOTLAND

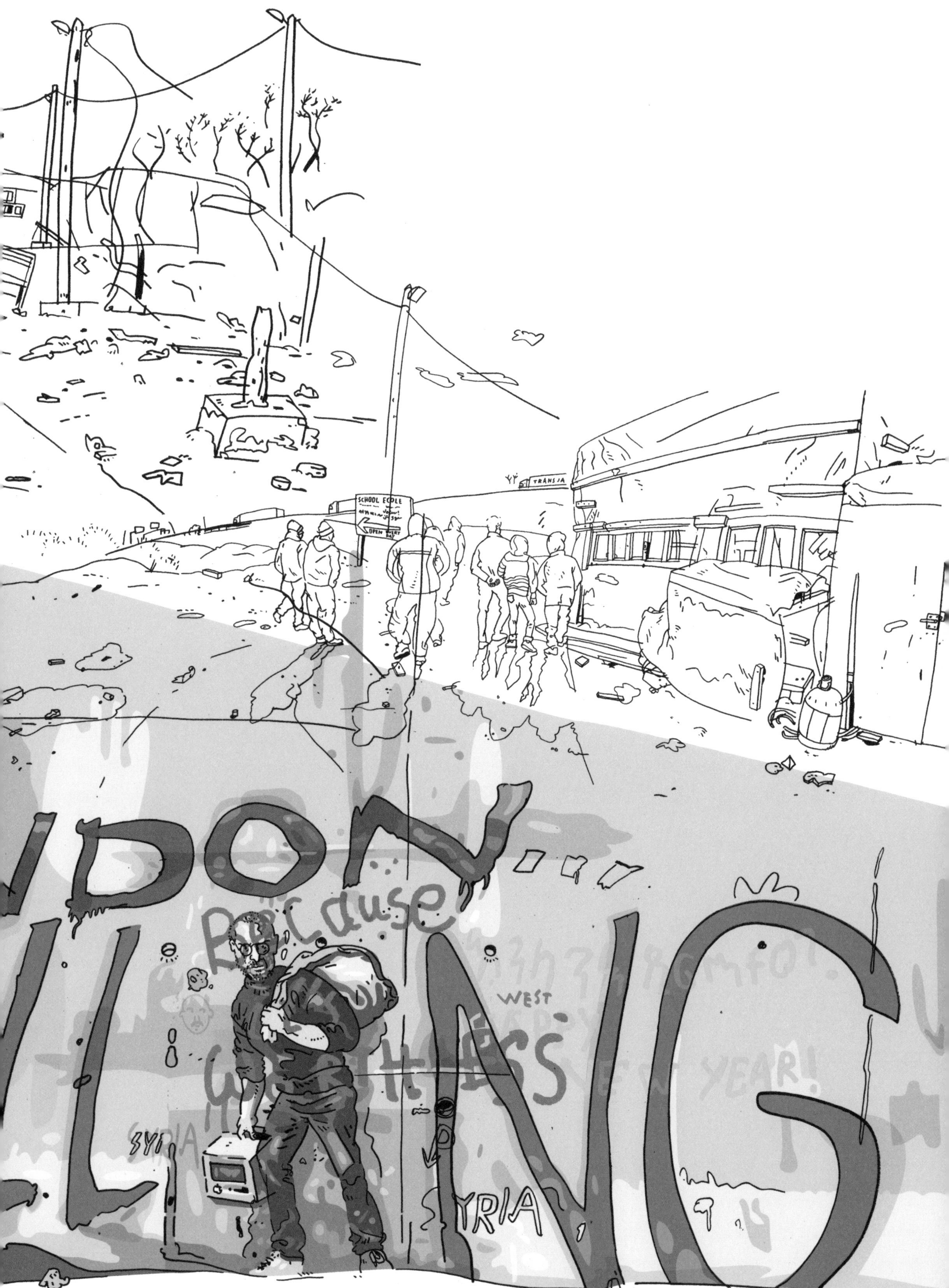
SCHOOL ECOLE
OPEN EVERY DAY
DON
Because
WEST
YEAR!
SYRIA
YRIA
NG

JOBS WAS BORN IN CALIFORNIA... HIS FATHER WAS A POLITICAL MIGRANT FROM THE SYRIAN CITY OF HOMS.

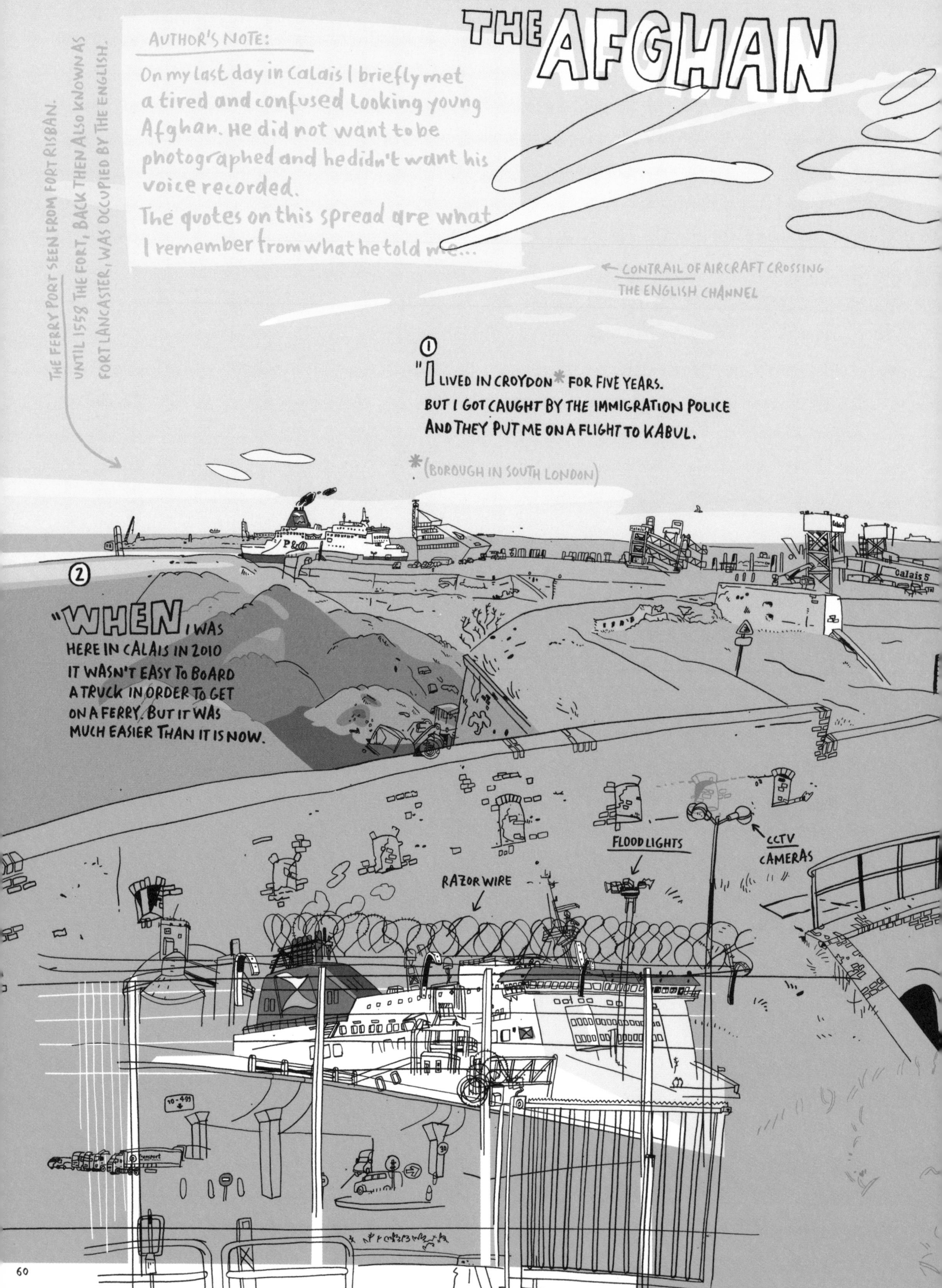
THE AFGHAN
AUTHOR'S NOTE:
On my last day in Calais I briefly met a tired and confused looking young Afghan. He did not want to be photographed and he didn't want his voice recorded.
The quotes on this spread are what I remember from what he told me...
THE FERRY PORT SEEN FROM FORT RISBAN.
UNTIL 1558 THE FORT, BACK THEN ALSO KNOWN AS FORT LANCASTER, WAS OCCUPIED BY THE ENGLISH.
← CONTRAIL OF AIRCRAFT CROSSING THE ENGLISH CHANNEL
① "I LIVED IN CROYDON* FOR FIVE YEARS. BUT I GOT CAUGHT BY THE IMMIGRATION POLICE AND THEY PUT ME ON A FLIGHT TO KABUL.
*(BOROUGH IN SOUTH LONDON)
P&O
Calais 5
② "WHEN I WAS HERE IN CALAIS IN 2010 IT WASN'T EASY TO BOARD A TRUCK IN ORDER TO GET ON A FERRY. BUT IT WAS MUCH EASIER THAN IT IS NOW.
FLOOD LIGHTS
CCTV CAMERAS
RAZOR WIRE
10-499
30

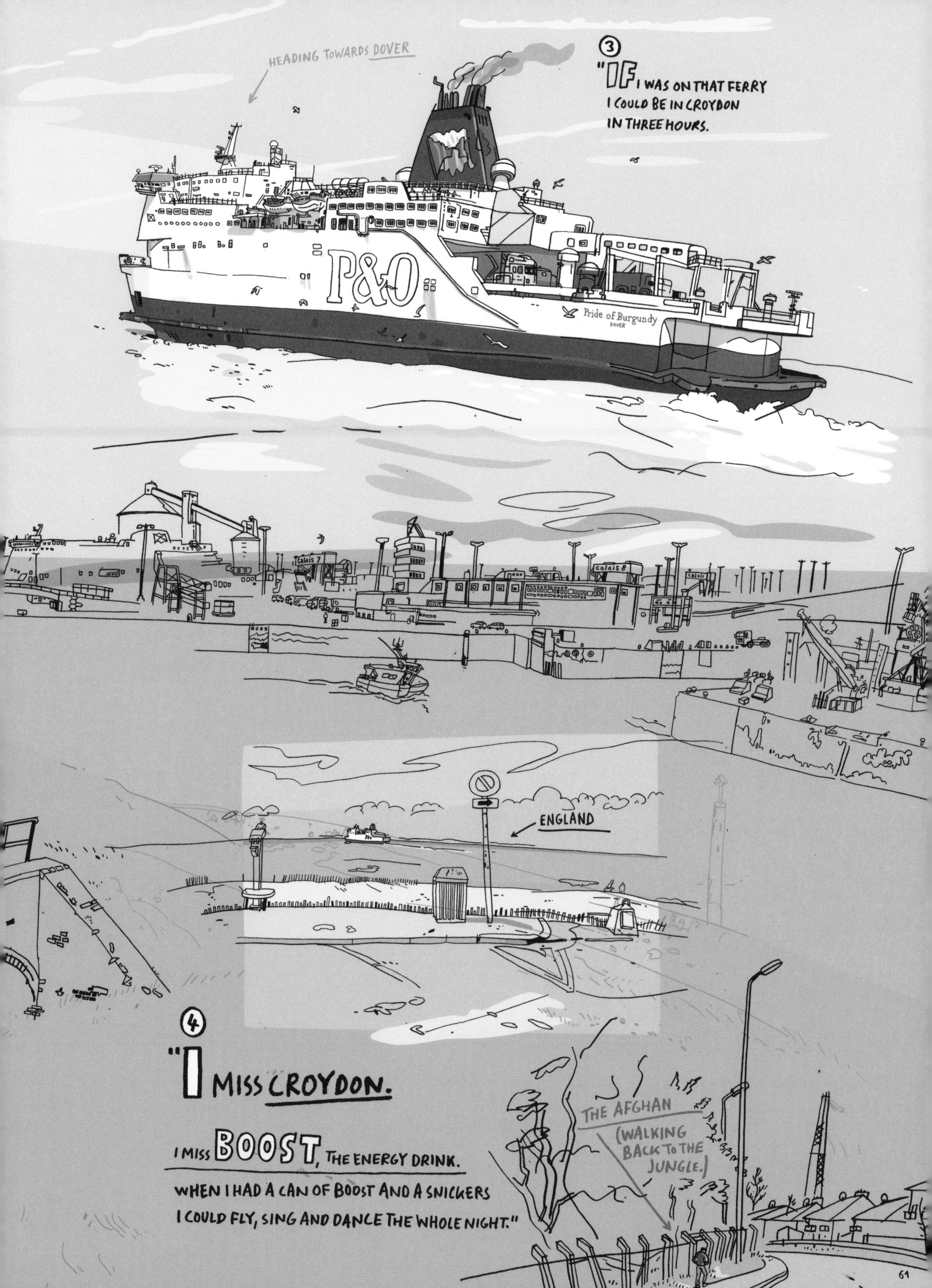

HEADING TOWARDS DOVER
③
"IF I WAS ON THAT FERRY
I COULD BE IN CROYDON
IN THREE HOURS.
P&O
Pride of Burgundy
DOVER
Calais 7
Calais 8
ENGLAND
④
"I MISS CROYDON.
I MISS BOOST, THE ENERGY DRINK.
WHEN I HAD A CAN OF BOOST AND A SNICKERS
I COULD FLY, SING AND DANCE THE WHOLE NIGHT."
THE AFGHAN
(WALKING BACK TO THE JUNGLE.)

ENGLAND

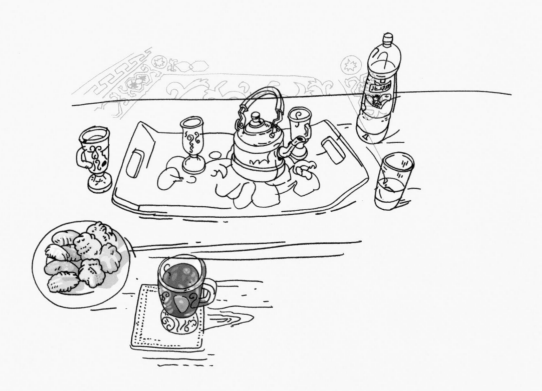

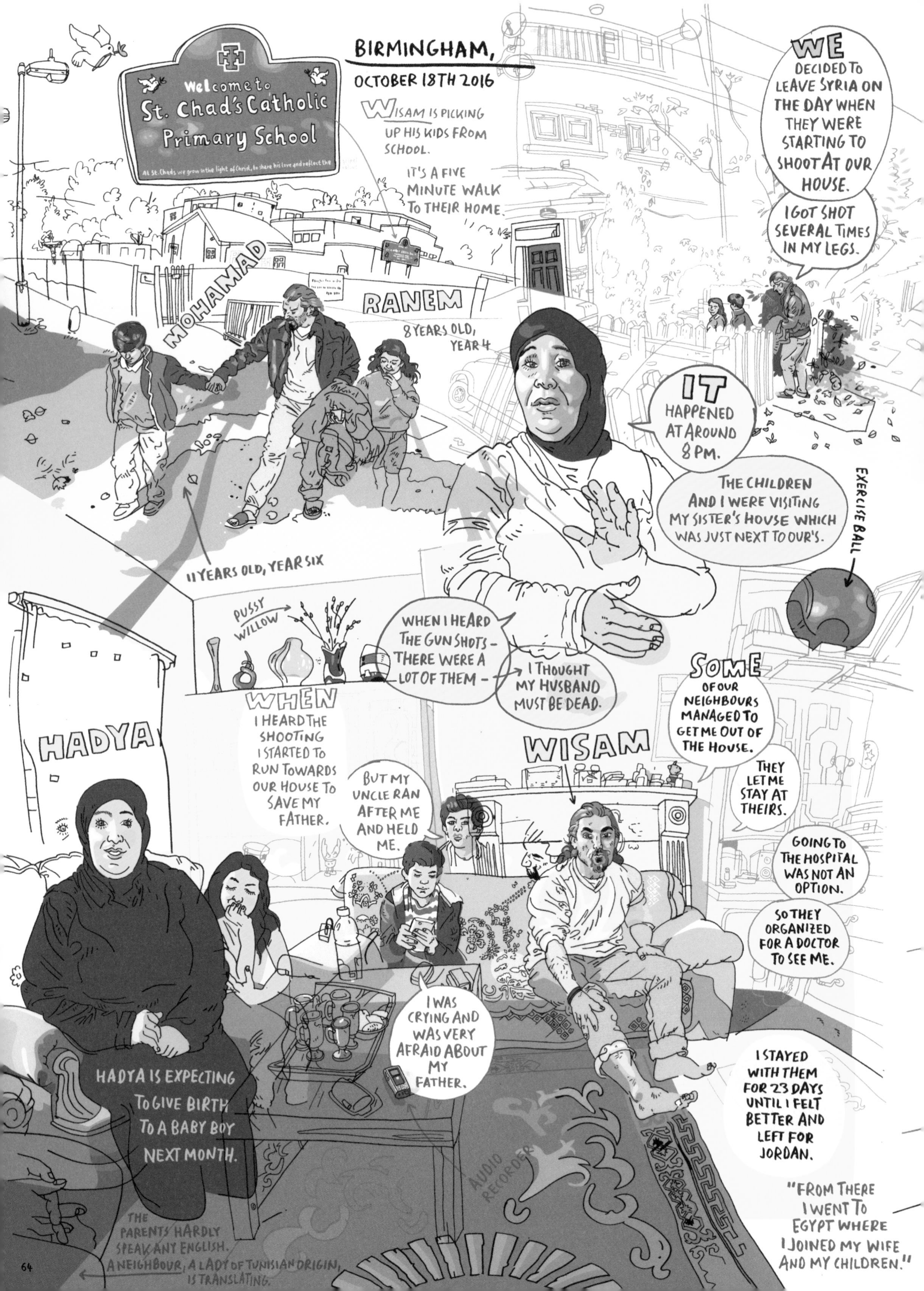

BIRMINGHAM,
OCTOBER 18TH 2016
Welcome to St. Chad's Catholic Primary School
At St. Chads we grow in the light of Christ, to share his love and reflect the
WISAM IS PICKING UP HIS KIDS FROM SCHOOL.
IT'S A FIVE MINUTE WALK TO THEIR HOME.
MOHAMAD
RANEM
8 YEARS OLD, YEAR 4
11 YEARS OLD, YEAR SIX
WE DECIDED TO LEAVE SYRIA ON THE DAY WHEN THEY WERE STARTING TO SHOOT AT OUR HOUSE.
I GOT SHOT SEVERAL TIMES IN MY LEGS.
IT HAPPENED AT AROUND 8 PM.
THE CHILDREN AND I WERE VISITING MY SISTER'S HOUSE WHICH WAS JUST NEXT TO OUR'S.
EXERCISE BALL
PUSSY WILLOW
WHEN I HEARD THE GUN SHOTS - THERE WERE A LOT OF THEM -
I THOUGHT MY HUSBAND MUST BE DEAD.
HADYA
WHEN I HEARD THE SHOOTING I STARTED TO RUN TOWARDS OUR HOUSE TO SAVE MY FATHER.
BUT MY UNCLE RAN AFTER ME AND HELD ME.
WISAM
SOME OF OUR NEIGHBOURS MANAGED TO GET ME OUT OF THE HOUSE.
THEY LET ME STAY AT THEIRS.
GOING TO THE HOSPITAL WAS NOT AN OPTION.
SO THEY ORGANIZED FOR A DOCTOR TO SEE ME.
I WAS CRYING AND WAS VERY AFRAID ABOUT MY FATHER.
I STAYED WITH THEM FOR 23 DAYS UNTIL I FELT BETTER AND LEFT FOR JORDAN.
HADYA IS EXPECTING TO GIVE BIRTH TO A BABY BOY NEXT MONTH.
AUDIO RECORDER
"FROM THERE I WENT TO EGYPT WHERE I JOINED MY WIFE AND MY CHILDREN."
THE PARENTS HARDLY SPEAK ANY ENGLISH. A NEIGHBOUR, A LADY OF TUNISIAN ORIGIN, IS TRANSLATING.

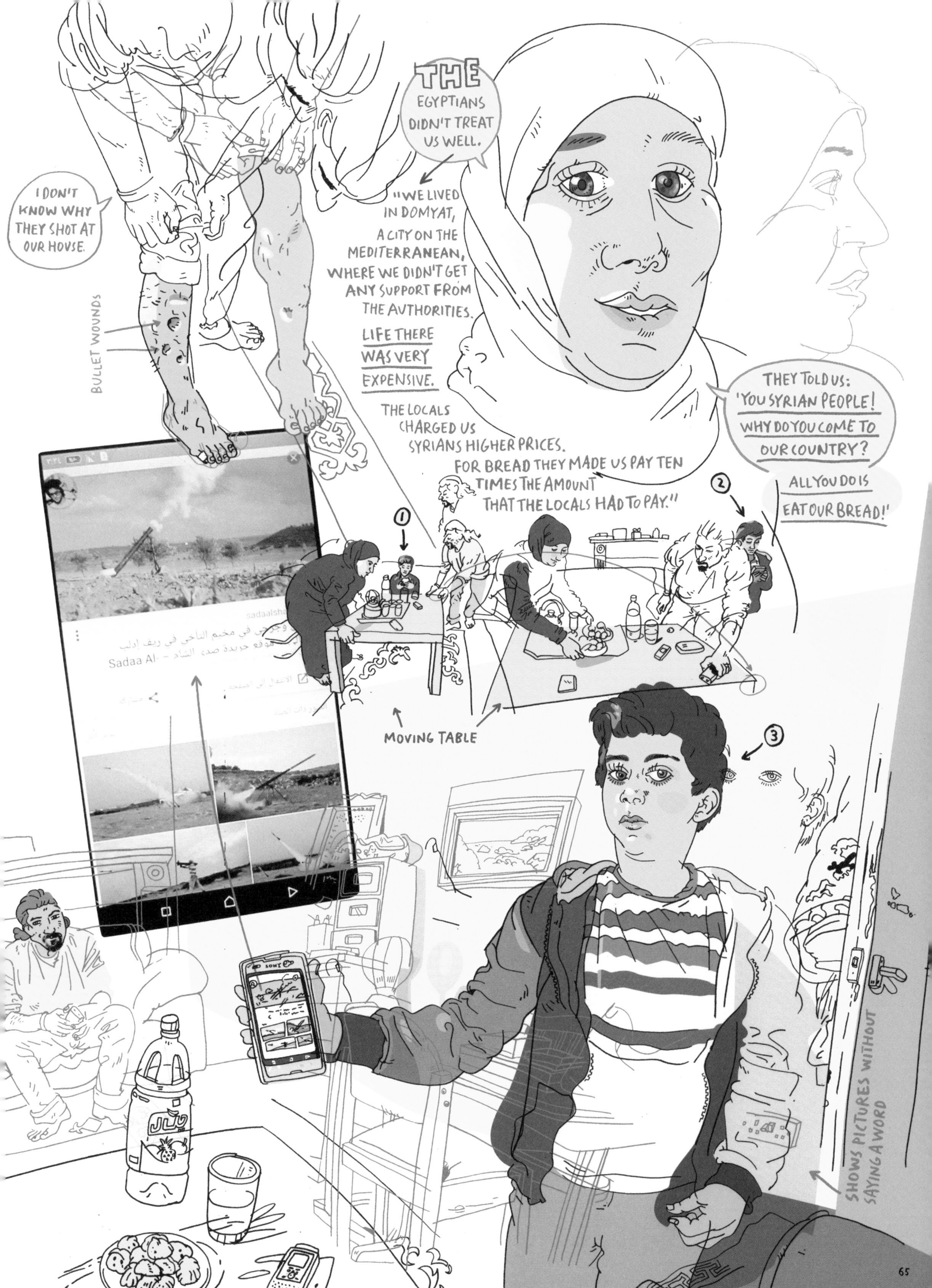

I DON'T KNOW WHY THEY SHOT AT OUR HOUSE.
BULLET WOUNDS
THE EGYPTIANS DIDN'T TREAT US WELL.
"WE LIVED IN DOMYAT, A CITY ON THE MEDITERRANEAN, WHERE WE DIDN'T GET ANY SUPPORT FROM THE AUTHORITIES.
LIFE THERE WAS VERY EXPENSIVE.
THE LOCALS CHARGED US SYRIANS HIGHER PRICES.
FOR BREAD THEY MADE US PAY TEN TIMES THE AMOUNT THAT THE LOCALS HAD TO PAY."
THEY TOLD US: 'YOU SYRIAN PEOPLE! WHY DO YOU COME TO OUR COUNTRY?
ALL YOU DO IS EAT OUR BREAD!'
1
2
3
MOVING TABLE
SONY
SHOWS PICTURES WITHOUT SAYING A WORD

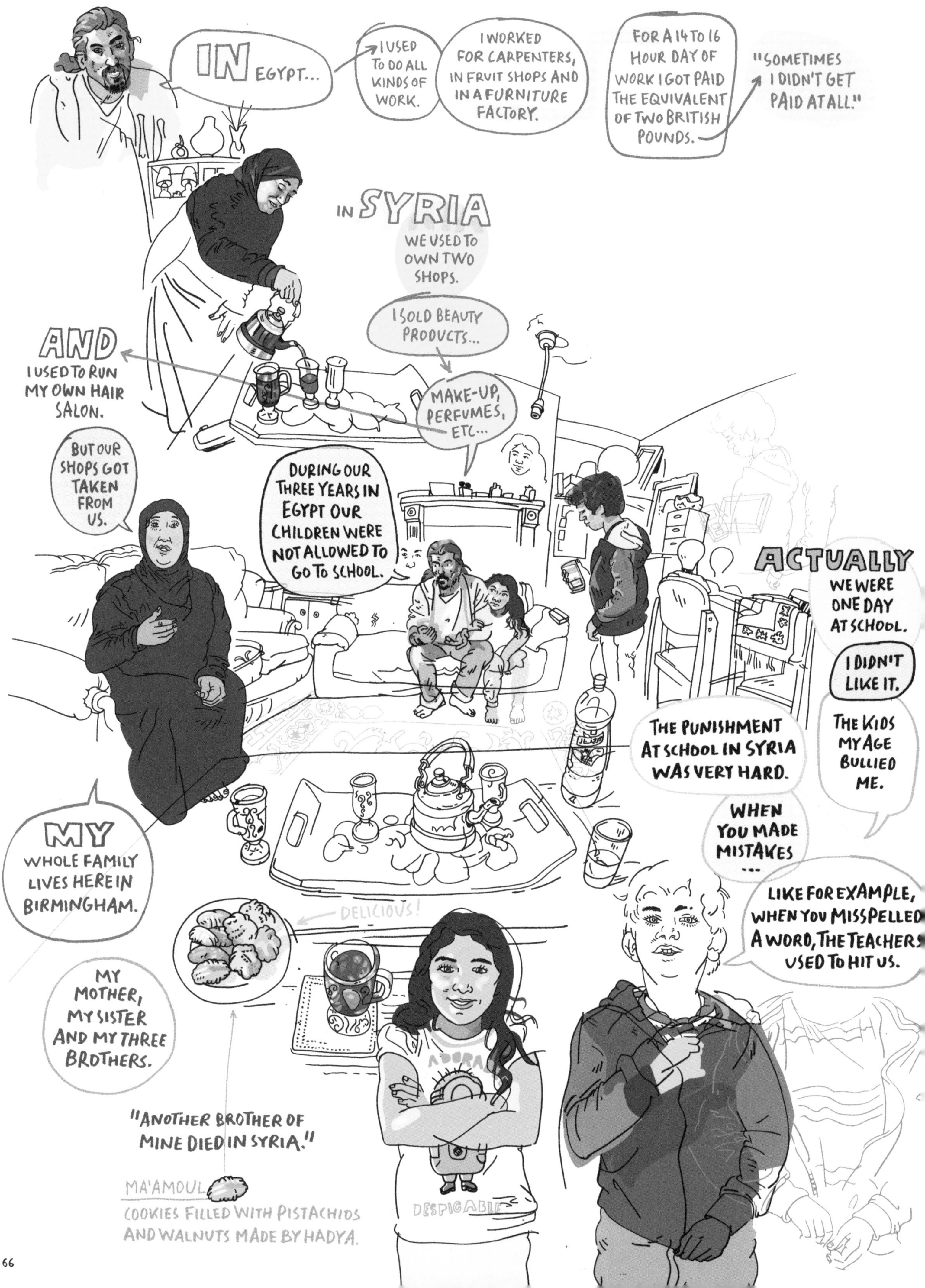
IN EGYPT...
I USED TO DO ALL KINDS OF WORK.
I WORKED FOR CARPENTERS, IN FRUIT SHOPS AND IN A FURNITURE FACTORY.
FOR A 14 TO 16 HOUR DAY OF WORK I GOT PAID THE EQUIVALENT OF TWO BRITISH POUNDS.
"SOMETIMES I DIDN'T GET PAID AT ALL."
IN SYRIA
WE USED TO OWN TWO SHOPS.
I SOLD BEAUTY PRODUCTS...
MAKE-UP, PERFUMES, ETC...
AND I USED TO RUN MY OWN HAIR SALON.
BUT OUR SHOPS GOT TAKEN FROM US.
DURING OUR THREE YEARS IN EGYPT OUR CHILDREN WERE NOT ALLOWED TO GO TO SCHOOL.
ACTUALLY WE WERE ONE DAY AT SCHOOL.
I DIDN'T LIKE IT.
THE KIDS MY AGE BULLIED ME.
THE PUNISHMENT AT SCHOOL IN SYRIA WAS VERY HARD.
WHEN YOU MADE MISTAKES ...
LIKE FOR EXAMPLE, WHEN YOU MISSPELLED A WORD, THE TEACHERS USED TO HIT US.
MY WHOLE FAMILY LIVES HERE IN BIRMINGHAM.
MY MOTHER, MY SISTER AND MY THREE BROTHERS.
"ANOTHER BROTHER OF MINE DIED IN SYRIA."
DELICIOUS!
MA'AMOUL
COOKIES FILLED WITH PISTACHIOS AND WALNUTS MADE BY HADYA.
ADORA
DESPICABLE

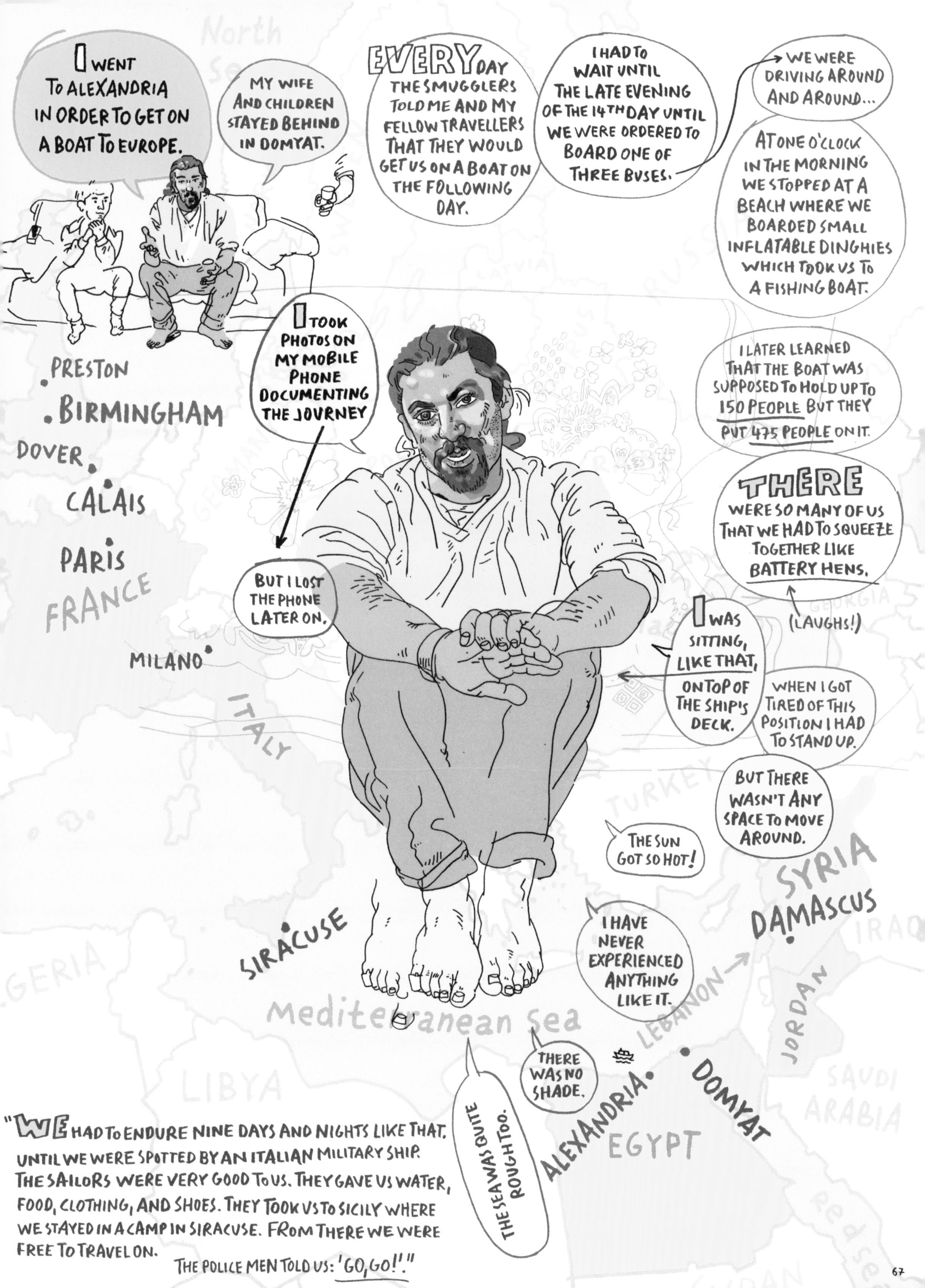
I WENT TO ALEXANDRIA IN ORDER TO GET ON A BOAT TO EUROPE.
MY WIFE AND CHILDREN STAYED BEHIND IN DOMYAT.
EVERY DAY THE SMUGGLERS TOLD ME AND MY FELLOW TRAVELLERS THAT THEY WOULD GET US ON A BOAT ON THE FOLLOWING DAY.
I HAD TO WAIT UNTIL THE LATE EVENING OF THE 14TH DAY UNTIL WE WERE ORDERED TO BOARD ONE OF THREE BUSES.
WE WERE DRIVING AROUND AND AROUND...
AT ONE O'CLOCK IN THE MORNING WE STOPPED AT A BEACH WHERE WE BOARDED SMALL INFLATABLE DINGHIES WHICH TOOK US TO A FISHING BOAT.
I TOOK PHOTOS ON MY MOBILE PHONE DOCUMENTING THE JOURNEY
BUT I LOST THE PHONE LATER ON.
I LATER LEARNED THAT THE BOAT WAS SUPPOSED TO HOLD UP TO 150 PEOPLE BUT THEY PUT 475 PEOPLE ON IT.
THERE WERE SO MANY OF US THAT WE HAD TO SQUEEZE TOGETHER LIKE BATTERY HENS.
(LAUGHS!)
I WAS SITTING, LIKE THAT, ON TOP OF THE SHIP'S DECK.
WHEN I GOT TIRED OF THIS POSITION I HAD TO STAND UP.
BUT THERE WASN'T ANY SPACE TO MOVE AROUND.
THE SUN GOT SO HOT!
I HAVE NEVER EXPERIENCED ANYTHING LIKE IT.
THERE WAS NO SHADE.
THE SEA WAS QUITE ROUGH TOO.
PRESTON
BIRMINGHAM
DOVER
CALAIS
PARIS
FRANCE
MILANO
ITALY
SIRACUSE
Mediterranean Sea
TURKEY
SYRIA
DAMASCUS
IRAQ
LEBANON
JORDAN
ALEXANDRIA
DOMYAT
EGYPT
LIBYA
SAUDI ARABIA
"WE HAD TO ENDURE NINE DAYS AND NIGHTS LIKE THAT. UNTIL WE WERE SPOTTED BY AN ITALIAN MILITARY SHIP. THE SAILORS WERE VERY GOOD TO US. THEY GAVE US WATER, FOOD, CLOTHING, AND SHOES. THEY TOOK US TO SICILY WHERE WE STAYED IN A CAMP IN SIRACUSE. FROM THERE WE WERE FREE TO TRAVEL ON.
THE POLICE MEN TOLD US: 'GO, GO!'."

HADYA: "I WAS EXTREMELY WORRIED. JUST AFTER WISAM WENT TO SEA TWO OTHER MIGRANT BOATS SANK ON THEIR WAY TO ITALY... AROUND 800 PEOPLE DROWNED. I THOUGHT THAT WISAM WAS ON BOARD ONE OF THESE BOATS. I DIDN'T DARE TO TELL OUR CHILDREN AS THEY WERE ALREADY TRAUMATIZED BY PREVIOUS EVENTS AND I DIDN'T WANT TO WORRY THEM AS WELL." **WISAM**: "I TOOK TRAINS TO MILAN AND FROM THERE TO PARIS. ON MY JOURNEY FROM ITALY TO FRANCE I SPENT MORE THAN £600 ON TRAIN TICKETS! I THINK I SPENT TOO MUCH... I WAS LOST." **HADYA**: "I HAD SOME GOLD JEWELLER[Y] THAT I SOLD. WE ALSO BORROWED MONEY TO PAY FOR WISAM'S JOURNEY." **WISAM**: "FROM PARIS I TRAVELLED ON TO CALAIS WHERE I WENT TO THE 'JUNGLE'. I DIDN'T LIKE THE PLACE... SO I WAS CAMPING OUT IN THE PORT AREA WHILST I WAS ATTEMPTING TO REACH GREAT BRITAIN. ONE DAY A COUPLE OF OTHER GUYS AND I PAID A SMUGGLER £4,000 EACH... IT WAS 'CHEAP' BACK THEN... NOW YOU WOULD HAVE TO PAY £7,000 TO £8,000 TO GET FROM CALAIS TO ENGLAND. THE GUY TOOK US TO A TRUCK AND SAID THAT THE TRUCK WAS SCHEDULED TO GO TO ENGLAND. HE OPENED THE DOORS AND LET US IN. IT WAS A REFRIGERATED TRAILER CARRYING BOXES OF CHOCOLATE. WE HID BEHIND THE BOXES AND THE SMUGGLER SHUT THE DOOR FROM THE OUTSIDE. BUT INSTEAD OF TAKING US TO ENGLAND THE TRUCK WENT TO BELGIUM. THERE WERE SEVERAL OTHER FAILED ATTEMPTS. BUT FINALLY ON THE 21ST DAY, THERE WERE THREE OF US, WE MANAGED TO GET IN A UK BOUND TRUCK. BUT THE DRIVER MUST HAVE SOMEHOW NOTICED US... HE OPENED THE DOOR AND DISCOVERED ONE OF US AND MADE HIM LEAVE THE TRAILER. BUT HE DIDN'T SEE US. AT THE FERRY PORT POLICE MEN ENTERED THE TRAILER. ONE OF THEM WAS ACTUALLY STANDING ON TOP OF THE BOX WE WERE HIDING IN WE WERE PUTTING OUR HANDS AND KNEES UP, LIKE THAT, TO SUPPORT THE BOX. THEY DID NOT DISCOVER US. ABOUT ONE AND A HALF HOURS DRIVE AFTER WE HAD ARRIVED IN DOVER MY FRIEND FELT UNWELL. WE BANGE[D] ON THE WALL NEXT TO THE DRIVER'S CABIN FOR ABOUT HALF AN HOUR UNTIL THE DRIVER STOPPED AND OPENED TH[E] DOOR. MY FIRST VIEW OF ENGLAND WAS THE SURPRISED TRUCKER. I SAID 'THANK YOU' TO HIM (LAUGHS WHEN HE SAYS THIS). BUT HE WAS JUST GESTICULATING, SHOOING US AWAY SAYING 'GO, GO, GO!'.

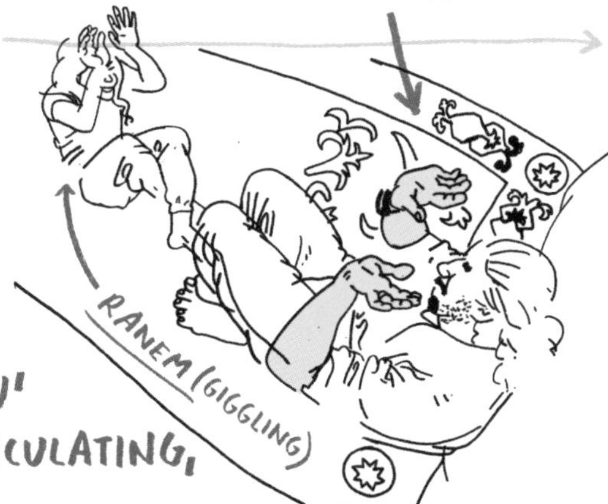
RANEM (GIGGLING)

HE LEFT US IN THE MIDDLE OF NOWHERE... THERE WAS LOTS OF GREEN. I WAS SO HAPPY TO HAVE FINALLY ARRIVED IN ENGLAND. WE THEN TRIED TO STOP SOME CARS ON THE ROAD BUT NOBODY STOPPED. SO WE WENT TO A HOUSE FURTHER UP THE ROAD. I TOLD THE PEOPLE THERE 'POLICE, POLICE... I AM ARAB, I AM SYRIAN...' I CROSSED MY WRISTS AS IF THEY WERE HAND CUFFED AND SAID: 'COME ON POLICE, POLICE...' ONE AND A HALF HOURS LATER THE POLICE CAME. THEY WERE VERY NICE AND TOOK US BACK TO DOVER WHERE THEY INTERVIEWED US. AFTERWARDS THEY DROVE US TO A HOSTEL IN LONDON, WHERE WE GOT ROOMS, A MEAL AND SOME MONEY. I THEN BOUGHT MYSELF A SIM CARD AND CALLED MY WIFE IN EGYPT."

THIS WAS ON THE 18TH OF MAY 2015.

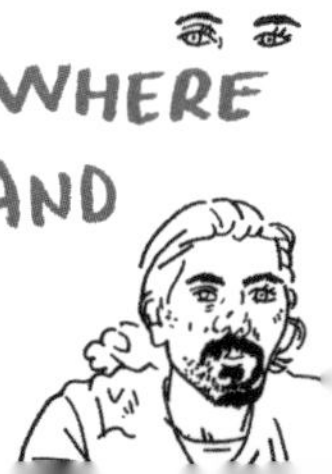

HADYA: "I WAS EXTREMELY HAPPY TO HEAR FROM HIM THAT HE ARRIVED SAFELY IN GREAT BRITAIN AND I GOT VERY EXCITED WITH THE PROSPECT OF JOINING HIM THERE SOON. OUR KIDS AND I ARRIVED IN BIRMINGHAM, VIA CAIRO AND ISTANBUL ON THE 22ND OF DECEMBER 2015. WE ARE VERY GRATEFUL TO THE RED CROSS WHO HELPED US OUT A LOT. THEY EVEN PAID FOR OUR TICKETS AS WE WERE OUT OF MONEY BY THEN. WHEN WE ARRIVED HERE THE COUNCIL PUT US UP IN A HOSTEL FOR SEVEN DAYS AND THEN THEY GAVE US THIS PLACE." **WISAM**: "BEFORE I WAS REUNITED WITH MY FAMILY I SPENT 14 DAYS IN LIVERPOOL AND IN PRESTON. I LIKED PRESTON A LOT... IT IS A GOOD PLACE... IT IS MUCH CALMER AND THE PEOPLE THERE WERE VERY GOOD." **HADYA**: "BUT I PREFER BIRMINGHAM BECAUSE MY WHOLE FAMILY LIVES HERE NOW." **WISAM**: "WE DON'T THINK THAT WE WILL GO BACK TO SYRIA ONE DAY... WE DON'T HAVE ANYTHING LEFT THERE NOW." **MOHAMAD**: "I AM NOT GOING TO GO BACK." **RANEM**: "I MISS MY AUNTS, THE SISTERS OF MY FATHER." (RANEM WAS 3 YEARS OLD WHEN SHE LEFT SYRIA). **MOHAMAD**: "I MISS OUR HOUSE IN SYRIA... I MISS PLAYING FOOTBALL AND TAG WITH MY OLD SCHOOL FRIENDS. BEFORE I CAME TO ENGLAND I DIDN'T REALLY KNOW ANYTHING ABOUT ENGLAND. I ONLY KNEW THAT MY FATHER WAS THERE AND THAT HE SAID THAT HE LIKED IT THERE AND THAT IT WAS A GOOD PLACE..." **WISAM**: "I CAN'T FIND WORK RIGHT NOW AS MY ENGLISH IS NOT GOOD ENOUGH." **MOHAMAD**: "I LIKE GOING TO SCHOOL IN BIRMINGHAM. I LEARN A LOT... I'VE GOT MANY FRIENDS. MY FAVOURITE SUBJECT IS PHYSICAL EDUCATION. I WANT TO BECOME THE CAPTAIN OF MY SCHOOL'S FOOTBALL TEAM."

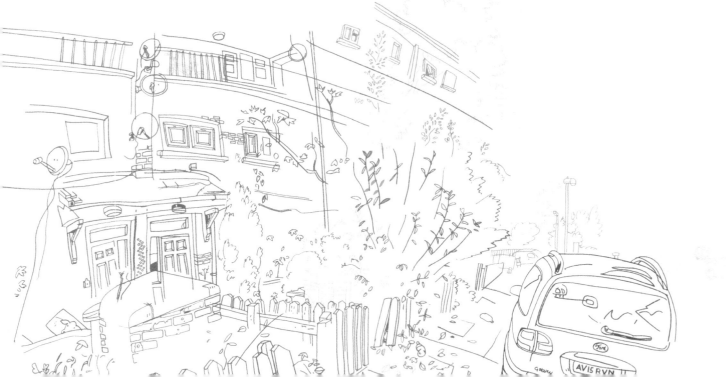

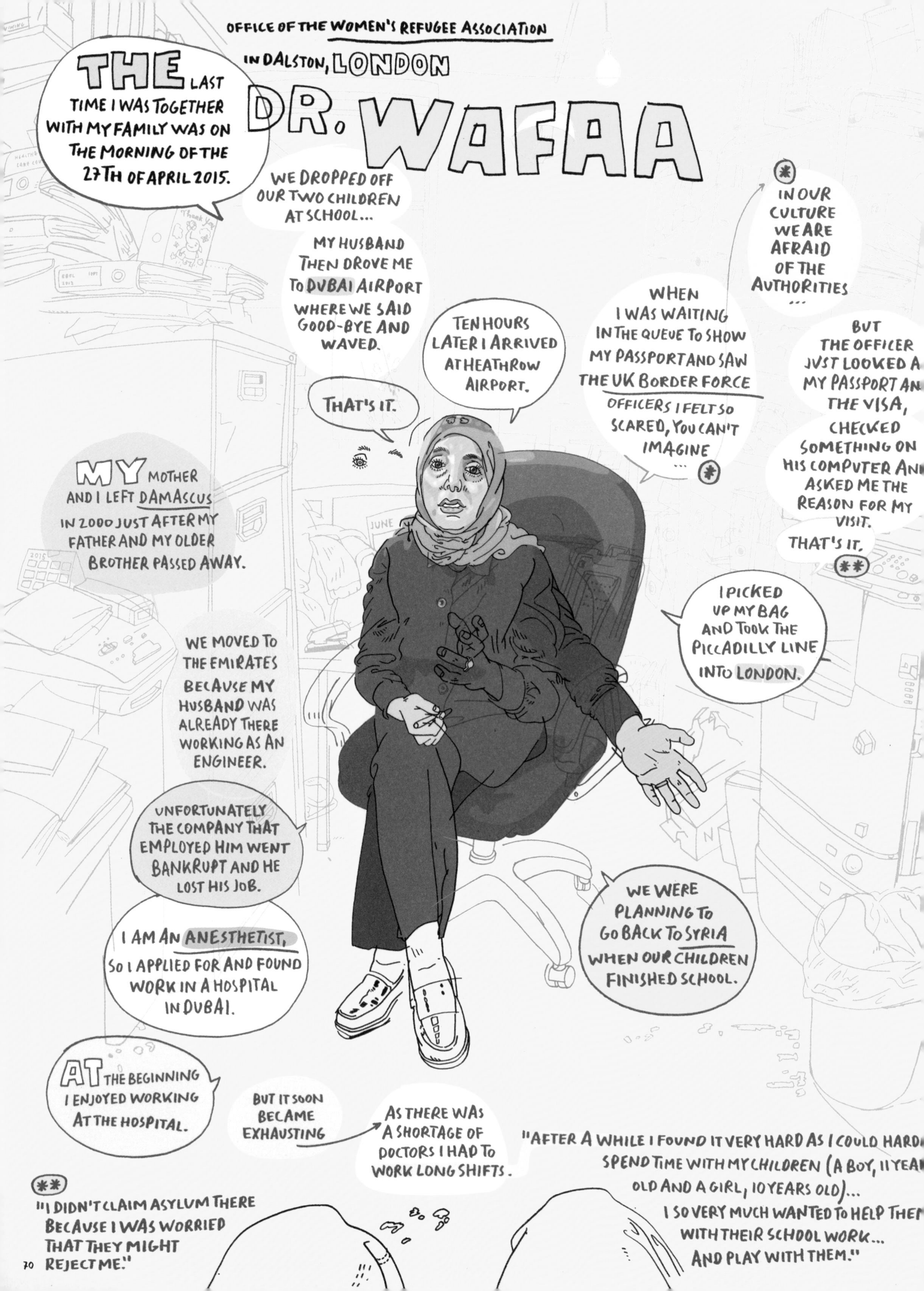

OFFICE OF THE WOMEN'S REFUGEE ASSOCIATION
IN DALSTON, LONDON
DR. WAFAA
THE LAST TIME I WAS TOGETHER WITH MY FAMILY WAS ON THE MORNING OF THE 27TH OF APRIL 2015.
WE DROPPED OFF OUR TWO CHILDREN AT SCHOOL...
MY HUSBAND THEN DROVE ME TO DUBAI AIRPORT WHERE WE SAID GOOD-BYE AND WAVED.
TEN HOURS LATER I ARRIVED AT HEATHROW AIRPORT.
THAT'S IT.
WHEN I WAS WAITING IN THE QUEUE TO SHOW MY PASSPORT AND SAW THE UK BORDER FORCE OFFICERS I FELT SO SCARED, YOU CAN'T IMAGINE ... (*)
(*) IN OUR CULTURE WE ARE AFRAID OF THE AUTHORITIES ...
BUT THE OFFICER JUST LOOKED A MY PASSPORT AN THE VISA, CHECKED SOMETHING ON HIS COMPUTER AN ASKED ME THE REASON FOR MY VISIT.
THAT'S IT. (**)
I PICKED UP MY BAG AND TOOK THE PICCADILLY LINE INTO LONDON.
MY MOTHER AND I LEFT DAMASCUS IN 2000 JUST AFTER MY FATHER AND MY OLDER BROTHER PASSED AWAY.
WE MOVED TO THE EMIRATES BECAUSE MY HUSBAND WAS ALREADY THERE WORKING AS AN ENGINEER.
UNFORTUNATELY THE COMPANY THAT EMPLOYED HIM WENT BANKRUPT AND HE LOST HIS JOB.
I AM AN ANESTHETIST, SO I APPLIED FOR AND FOUND WORK IN A HOSPITAL IN DUBAI.
WE WERE PLANNING TO GO BACK TO SYRIA WHEN OUR CHILDREN FINISHED SCHOOL.
AT THE BEGINNING I ENJOYED WORKING AT THE HOSPITAL.
BUT IT SOON BECAME EXHAUSTING
AS THERE WAS A SHORTAGE OF DOCTORS I HAD TO WORK LONG SHIFTS.
"AFTER A WHILE I FOUND IT VERY HARD AS I COULD HARD SPEND TIME WITH MY CHILDREN (A BOY, 11 YEA OLD AND A GIRL, 10 YEARS OLD)... I SO VERY MUCH WANTED TO HELP THEM WITH THEIR SCHOOL WORK... AND PLAY WITH THEM."
(**) "I DIDN'T CLAIM ASYLUM THERE BECAUSE I WAS WORRIED THAT THEY MIGHT REJECT ME."

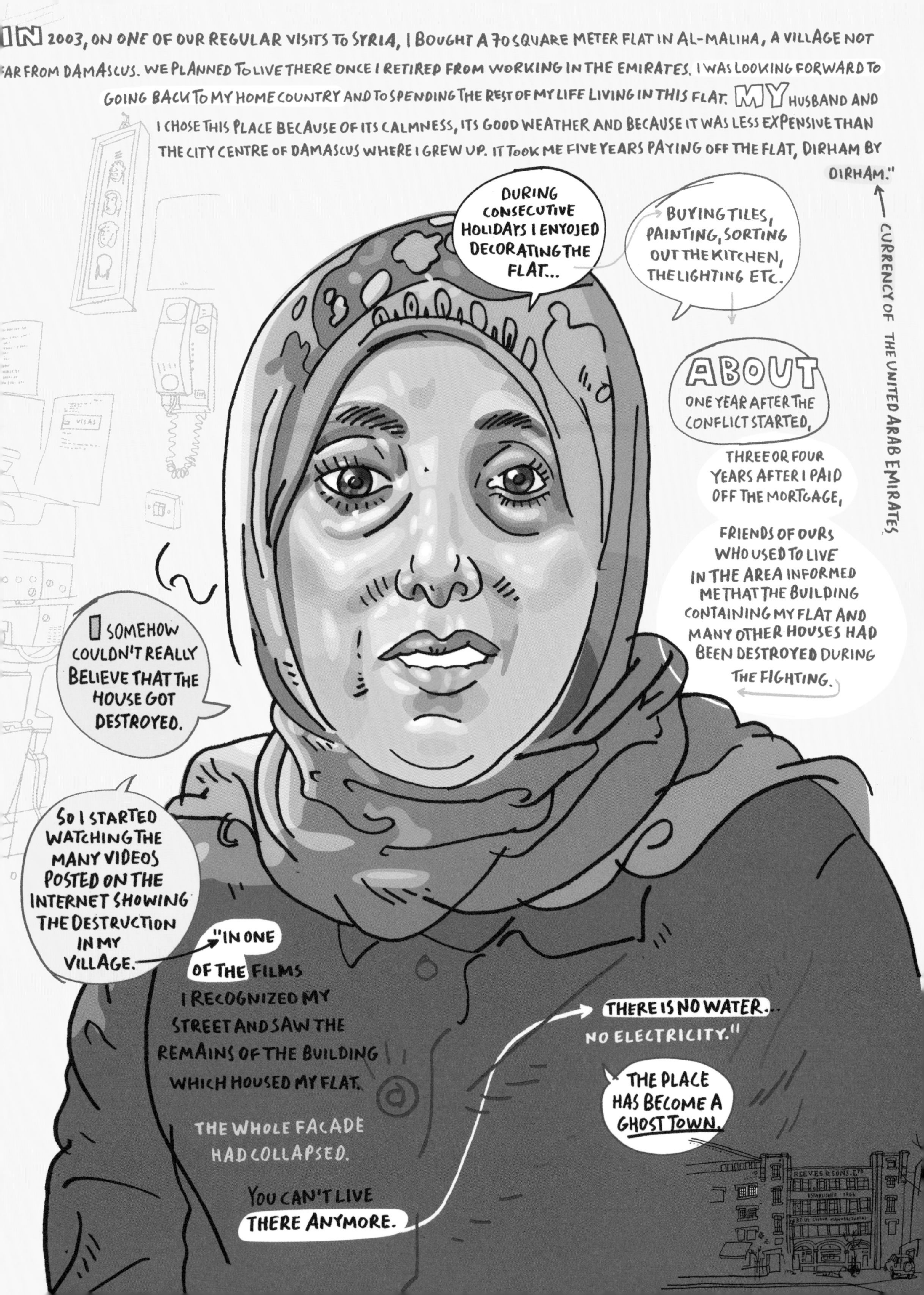
"IN 2003, ON ONE OF OUR REGULAR VISITS TO SYRIA, I BOUGHT A 70 SQUARE METER FLAT IN AL-MALIHA, A VILLAGE NOT FAR FROM DAMASCUS. WE PLANNED TO LIVE THERE ONCE I RETIRED FROM WORKING IN THE EMIRATES. I WAS LOOKING FORWARD TO GOING BACK TO MY HOME COUNTRY AND TO SPENDING THE REST OF MY LIFE LIVING IN THIS FLAT. MY HUSBAND AND I CHOSE THIS PLACE BECAUSE OF ITS CALMNESS, ITS GOOD WEATHER AND BECAUSE IT WAS LESS EXPENSIVE THAN THE CITY CENTRE OF DAMASCUS WHERE I GREW UP. IT TOOK ME FIVE YEARS PAYING OFF THE FLAT, DIRHAM BY DIRHAM."
CURRENCY OF THE UNITED ARAB EMIRATES
DURING CONSECUTIVE HOLIDAYS I ENYOJED DECORATING THE FLAT...
BUYING TILES, PAINTING, SORTING OUT THE KITCHEN, THE LIGHTING ETC.
ABOUT ONE YEAR AFTER THE CONFLICT STARTED,
THREE OR FOUR YEARS AFTER I PAID OFF THE MORTGAGE,
FRIENDS OF OURS WHO USED TO LIVE IN THE AREA INFORMED ME THAT THE BUILDING CONTAINING MY FLAT AND MANY OTHER HOUSES HAD BEEN DESTROYED DURING THE FIGHTING.
I SOMEHOW COULDN'T REALLY BELIEVE THAT THE HOUSE GOT DESTROYED.
SO I STARTED WATCHING THE MANY VIDEOS POSTED ON THE INTERNET SHOWING THE DESTRUCTION IN MY VILLAGE.
"IN ONE OF THE FILMS I RECOGNIZED MY STREET AND SAW THE REMAINS OF THE BUILDING WHICH HOUSED MY FLAT.
THE WHOLE FACADE HAD COLLAPSED.
YOU CAN'T LIVE THERE ANYMORE.
THERE IS NO WATER... NO ELECTRICITY."
THE PLACE HAS BECOME A GHOST TOWN.
VISAS

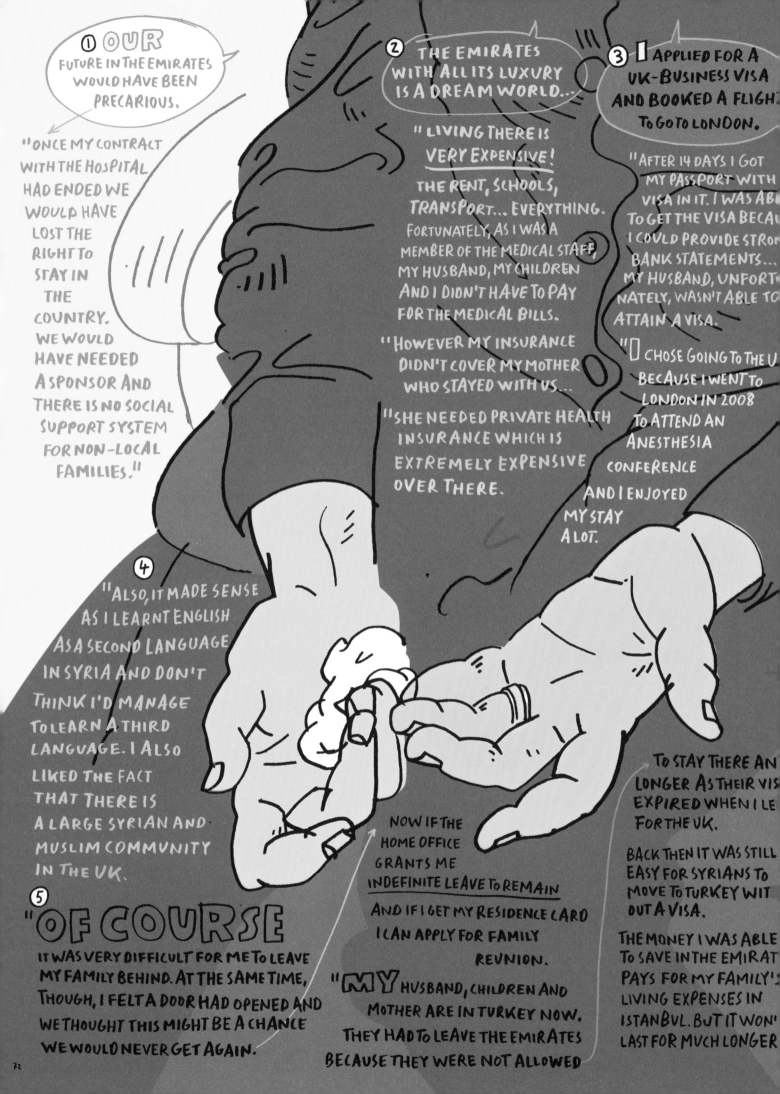

① **OUR** FUTURE IN THE EMIRATES WOULD HAVE BEEN PRECARIOUS.

"ONCE MY CONTRACT WITH THE HOSPITAL HAD ENDED WE WOULD HAVE LOST THE RIGHT TO STAY IN THE COUNTRY. WE WOULD HAVE NEEDED A SPONSOR AND THERE IS NO SOCIAL SUPPORT SYSTEM FOR NON-LOCAL FAMILIES."

② THE EMIRATES WITH ALL ITS LUXURY IS A DREAM WORLD...

"LIVING THERE IS VERY EXPENSIVE! THE RENT, SCHOOLS, TRANSPORT... EVERYTHING. FORTUNATELY, AS I WAS A MEMBER OF THE MEDICAL STAFF, MY HUSBAND, MY CHILDREN AND I DIDN'T HAVE TO PAY FOR THE MEDICAL BILLS.

"HOWEVER MY INSURANCE DIDN'T COVER MY MOTHER WHO STAYED WITH US...

"SHE NEEDED PRIVATE HEALTH INSURANCE WHICH IS EXTREMELY EXPENSIVE OVER THERE.

③ **I** APPLIED FOR A UK-BUSINESS VISA AND BOOKED A FLIGHT TO GO TO LONDON.

"AFTER 14 DAYS I GOT MY PASSPORT WITH VISA IN IT. I WAS ABLE TO GET THE VISA BECAUSE I COULD PROVIDE STRONG BANK STATEMENTS... MY HUSBAND, UNFORTUNATELY, WASN'T ABLE TO ATTAIN A VISA.

"I CHOSE GOING TO THE UK BECAUSE I WENT TO LONDON IN 2008 TO ATTEND AN ANESTHESIA CONFERENCE AND I ENJOYED MY STAY A LOT.

④ "ALSO, IT MADE SENSE AS I LEARNT ENGLISH AS A SECOND LANGUAGE IN SYRIA AND DON'T THINK I'D MANAGE TO LEARN A THIRD LANGUAGE. I ALSO LIKED THE FACT THAT THERE IS A LARGE SYRIAN AND MUSLIM COMMUNITY IN THE UK.

⑤ "OF COURSE IT WAS VERY DIFFICULT FOR ME TO LEAVE MY FAMILY BEHIND. AT THE SAME TIME, THOUGH, I FELT A DOOR HAD OPENED AND WE THOUGHT THIS MIGHT BE A CHANCE WE WOULD NEVER GET AGAIN.

NOW IF THE HOME OFFICE GRANTS ME INDEFINITE LEAVE TO REMAIN AND IF I GET MY RESIDENCE CARD I CAN APPLY FOR FAMILY REUNION.

"MY HUSBAND, CHILDREN AND MOTHER ARE IN TURKEY NOW. THEY HAD TO LEAVE THE EMIRATES BECAUSE THEY WERE NOT ALLOWED

TO STAY THERE ANY LONGER AS THEIR VISA EXPIRED WHEN I LEFT FOR THE UK.

BACK THEN IT WAS STILL EASY FOR SYRIANS TO MOVE TO TURKEY WITHOUT A VISA.

THE MONEY I WAS ABLE TO SAVE IN THE EMIRATES PAYS FOR MY FAMILY'S LIVING EXPENSES IN ISTANBUL. BUT IT WON'T LAST FOR MUCH LONGER

6 I AM IN CONTACT WITH MY FAMILY VIA SKYPE.

[I] CAN'T IMAGINE A DAY WITHOUT SEEING THEM TWICE AT LEAST. I FIND IT VERY DIFFICULT TO TALK WITH MY CHILDREN. SOMETIMES IT IS NOT POSSIBLE AS THEY WOULD RATHER PLAY VIDEO GAMES, CAN YOU IMAGINE? WHEN THEY DO TALK WITH ME THEY START TO TELL ME HOW MUCH THEY MISS ME AND THEY EXPRESS THEIR FRUSTRATION ABOUT OUR SEPARATION UNTIL THEY START CRYING. I DON'T WANT THEM TO CRY ANYMORE SO I TRY NOT TO DIG TOO DEEP INTO THEIR EMOTIONS... I TRY NOT TO BE TOO AFFECTIONATE WITH THEM. OTHERWISE THEY WILL START ASKING ME AGAIN WHEN THEY WILL BE WITH ME NEXT... 'WHEN?! PLEASE GIVE ME A DATE.' I CAN'T GIVE THEM A DATE. MY DAUGHTER ACCUSED ME OF LYING TO HER. IN THE PAST I TOLD HER THAT, MAYBE, WE WILL BE REUNITED IN TWO OR THREE MONTHS... BUT WHEN THE TIME PASSED IT STILL HADN'T HAPPENED...

[I] AM IN CONTACT WITH THE HOME OFFICE THROUGH MY MP RUPA HUQ... BUT THEY REPLIED THAT NO DECISION HAS BEEN MADE YET AND THAT THEY CAN'T GIVE ME ANY INFORMATION ABOUT WHEN THEY WILL BE ABLE TO MAKE A DECISION. I DON'T KNOW WHAT THEY ARE WAITING FOR... WHAT IS STOPPING THEM? MY CHILDREN NEED ME. MY DAUGHTER, I THINK, IS STARTING TO GET INTO PUBERTY... I TRY NOT TO THINK TOO MUCH ABOUT IT. I AM TRYING TO FOCUS ON IMPROVING MY ENGLISH SKILLS.

7 "[I] DON'T KNOW IF I'VE GOT THE RIGHT TO COMPLAIN. WHEN I HEAR OTHER PEOPLE'S STORIES I THINK MY STORY IS TRIVIAL. THERE ARE SO MANY PARENTS WHO LOST THEIR CHILDREN AND SO MANY CHILDREN BECAME ORPHANS.

SO I TRY NOT TO COMPLAIN, TO STAY QUIET AND TO BE PATIENT... I PRAY.

"MY CHILDREN SPEAK ENGLISH... AMERICAN ENGLISH! THEY WENT TO SCHOOLS WHERE THEY WERE TAUGHT BILINGUALLY. I WAS THINKING THAT MY CHILDREN HAVE NO IDENTITY... THEY WERE BORN IN THE EMIRATES AND DON'T SPEAK ARABIC WITH A DAMASCENE ACCENT... BUT NEITHER DO THEY SPEAK WITH AN EMIRATES ACCENT... AND NOW THEY ARE IN A TURKISH SCHOOL. LUCKILY THERE ARE MANY OTHER CHILDREN FROM SYRIA, IN FACT ALL THEIR FRIENDS ARE FROM DAMASCUS. THIS IS VERY COMFORTING FOR ME. MY CHILDREN KNOW NOW THAT THEY ARE SYRIAN. BEFORE, BEING SYRIAN, WAS JUST A VAGUE CONCEPT FOR THEM.

"[I] AM DOING VOLUNTARY WORK AT THE GREAT ORMOND STREET HOSPITAL ON A WARD, WHERE THE PATIENTS (CHILDREN) AND THEIR ACCOMPANYING MUMS ARE FROM OVERSEAS, MAINLY FROM ARABIC COUNTRIES. AT THE MOMENT I AM SUPPORTING A MUM WHOSE FOUR-MONTH-OLD CHILD IS RECEIVING CANCER TREATMENT. SO, IF THE MOTHER NEEDS TO TAKE A BREAK OR NEEDS TO HAVE A REST I LOOK AFTER HER BABY... I HOLD IT, FEED IT... CUDDLE IT.

"IDEALLY I WOULD LIKE TO WORK AS A DOCTOR IN THE UK... BUT I DON'T KNOW IF THIS WILL EVER BE POSSIBLE. THERE ARE MANY BARRIERS LIKE GETTING MY CERTIFICATE RECOGNIZED, THE LANGUAGE, THE TRAINING... I AM WORKING ON IT... I AM IN A BAD EMOTIONAL AND PHYSICAL SITUATION BUT I NEED TO BE STRONG."

GERMANY

IMS

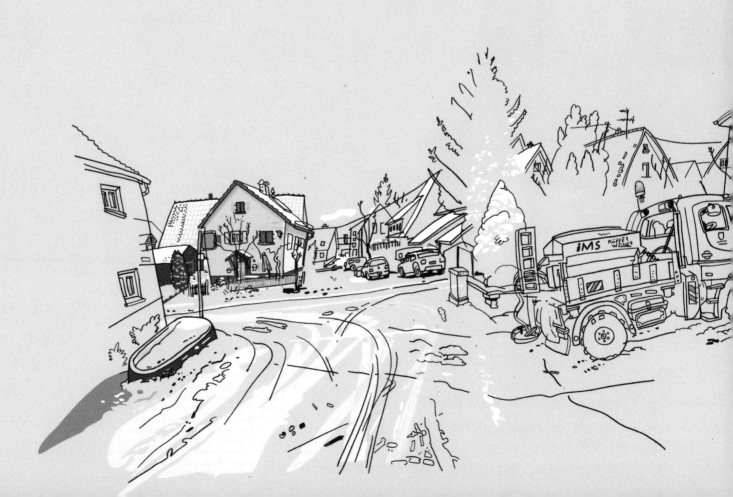

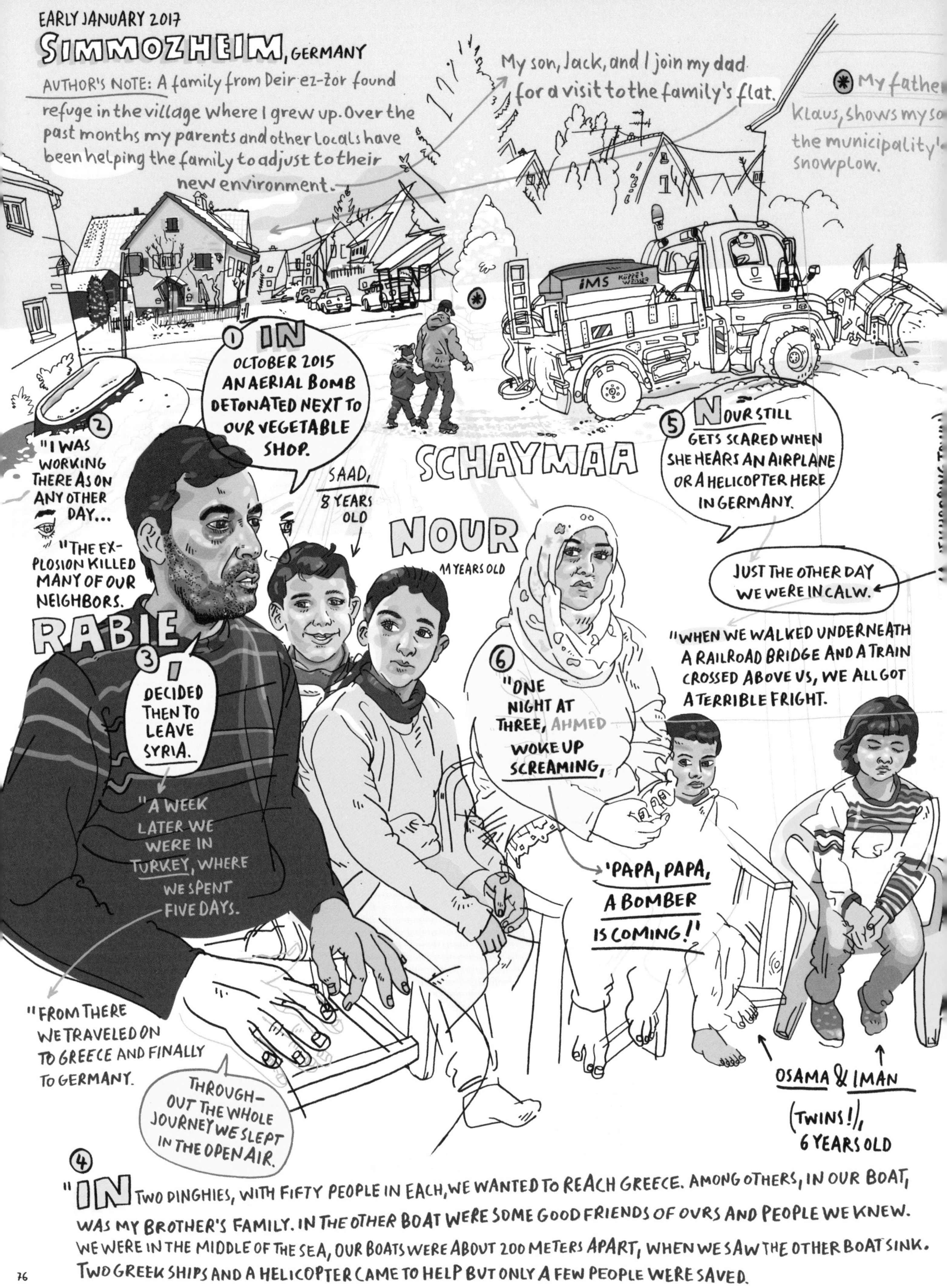
EARLY JANUARY 2017
SIMMOZHEIM, GERMANY
AUTHOR'S NOTE: A family from Deir ez-Zor found refuge in the village where I grew up. Over the past months my parents and other locals have been helping the family to adjust to their new environment.
My son, Jack, and I join my dad for a visit to the family's flat.
My fathe
Klaus, shows my so
the municipality'
snowplow.
IMS
① IN OCTOBER 2015 AN AERIAL BOMB DETONATED NEXT TO OUR VEGETABLE SHOP.
② "I WAS WORKING THERE AS ON ANY OTHER DAY...
"THE EXPLOSION KILLED MANY OF OUR NEIGHBORS.
RABIE
SAAD, 8 YEARS OLD
NOUR 11 YEARS OLD
SCHAYMAA
③ I DECIDED THEN TO LEAVE SYRIA.
"A WEEK LATER WE WERE IN TURKEY, WHERE WE SPENT FIVE DAYS.
"FROM THERE WE TRAVELED ON TO GREECE AND FINALLY TO GERMANY.
THROUGHOUT THE WHOLE JOURNEY WE SLEPT IN THE OPEN AIR.
⑤ NOUR STILL GETS SCARED WHEN SHE HEARS AN AIRPLANE OR A HELICOPTER HERE IN GERMANY.
JUST THE OTHER DAY WE WERE IN CALW.
"WHEN WE WALKED UNDERNEATH A RAILROAD BRIDGE AND A TRAIN CROSSED ABOVE US, WE ALL GOT A TERRIBLE FRIGHT.
⑥ "ONE NIGHT AT THREE, AHMED WOKE UP SCREAMING,
'PAPA, PAPA, A BOMBER IS COMING!'
OSAMA & IMAN (TWINS!), 6 YEARS OLD
④ "IN TWO DINGHIES, WITH FIFTY PEOPLE IN EACH, WE WANTED TO REACH GREECE. AMONG OTHERS, IN OUR BOAT, WAS MY BROTHER'S FAMILY. IN THE OTHER BOAT WERE SOME GOOD FRIENDS OF OURS AND PEOPLE WE KNEW. WE WERE IN THE MIDDLE OF THE SEA, OUR BOATS WERE ABOUT 200 METERS APART, WHEN WE SAW THE OTHER BOAT SINK. TWO GREEK SHIPS AND A HELICOPTER CAME TO HELP BUT ONLY A FEW PEOPLE WERE SAVED.

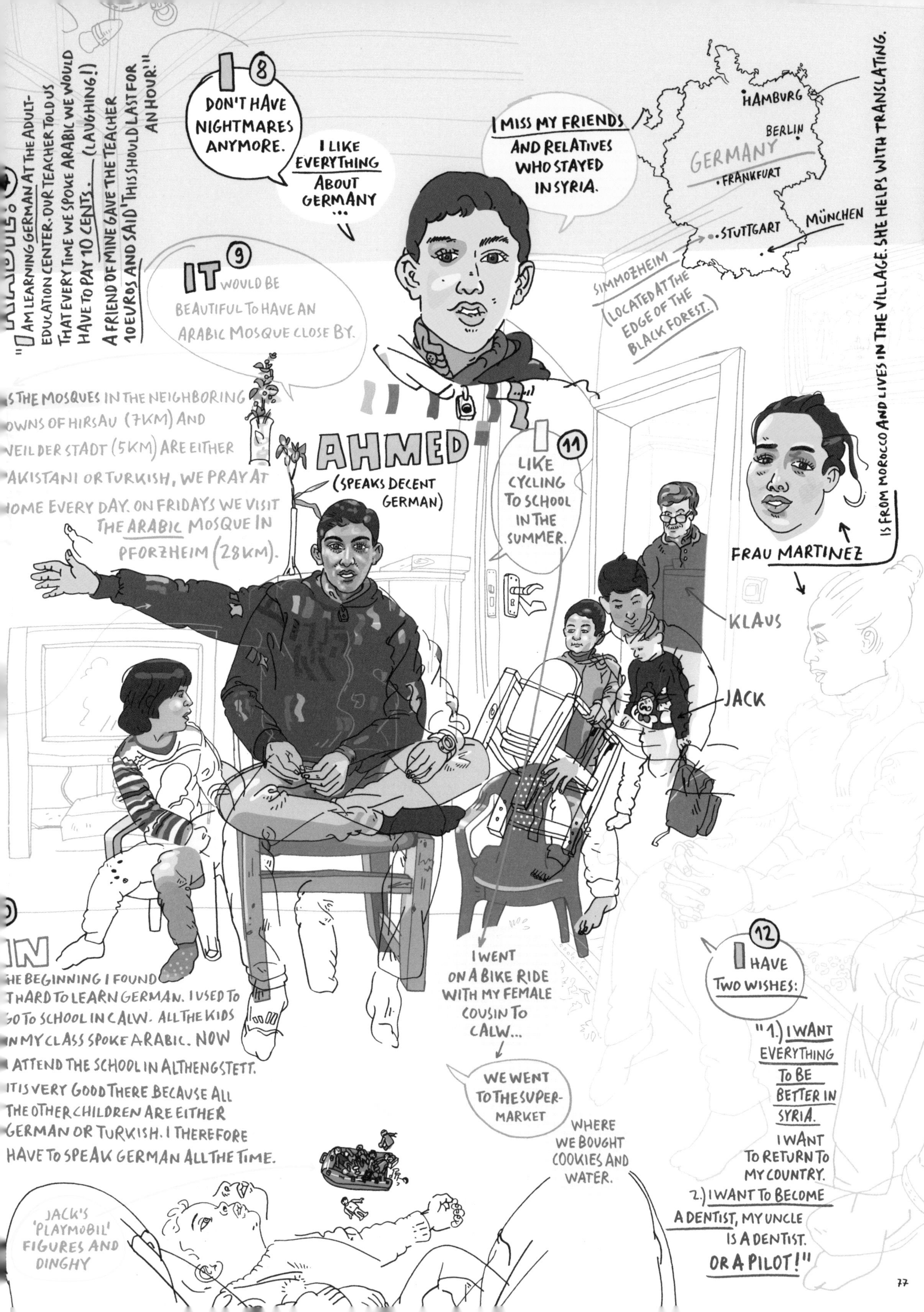
"I AM LEARNING GERMAN AT THE ADULT-EDUCATION CENTER. OUR TEACHER TOLD US THAT EVERY TIME WE SPOKE ARABIC WE WOULD HAVE TO PAY 10 CENTS. (LAUGHING!)
A FRIEND OF MINE GAVE THE TEACHER 10 EUROS AND SAID 'THIS SHOULD LAST FOR AN HOUR.'"
8
I DON'T HAVE NIGHTMARES ANYMORE.
I LIKE EVERYTHING ABOUT GERMANY ...
I MISS MY FRIENDS AND RELATIVES WHO STAYED IN SYRIA.
HAMBURG
BERLIN
GERMANY
FRANKFURT
STUTTGART
MÜNCHEN
SIMMOZHEIM (LOCATED AT THE EDGE OF THE BLACK FOREST.)
9
IT WOULD BE BEAUTIFUL TO HAVE AN ARABIC MOSQUE CLOSE BY.
S THE MOSQUES IN THE NEIGHBORING OWNS OF HIRSAU (7KM) AND VEIL DER STADT (5KM) ARE EITHER AKISTANI OR TURKISH, WE PRAY AT IOME EVERY DAY. ON FRIDAYS WE VISIT THE ARABIC MOSQUE IN PFORZHEIM (28KM).
AHMED
(SPEAKS DECENT GERMAN)
11
I LIKE CYCLING TO SCHOOL IN THE SUMMER.
IS FROM MOROCCO AND LIVES IN THE VILLAGE. SHE HELPS WITH TRANSLATING.
FRAU MARTINEZ
KLAUS
JACK
IN
HE BEGINNING I FOUND T HARD TO LEARN GERMAN. I USED TO GO TO SCHOOL IN CALW. ALL THE KIDS N MY CLASS SPOKE ARABIC. NOW ATTEND THE SCHOOL IN ALTHENGSTETT. IT IS VERY GOOD THERE BECAUSE ALL THE OTHER CHILDREN ARE EITHER GERMAN OR TURKISH. I THEREFORE HAVE TO SPEAK GERMAN ALL THE TIME.
I WENT ON A BIKE RIDE WITH MY FEMALE COUSIN TO CALW...
WE WENT TO THE SUPERMARKET
WHERE WE BOUGHT COOKIES AND WATER.
12
I HAVE TWO WISHES:
"1.) I WANT EVERYTHING TO BE BETTER IN SYRIA. I WANT TO RETURN TO MY COUNTRY.
2.) I WANT TO BECOME A DENTIST, MY UNCLE IS A DENTIST. OR A PILOT!"
JACK'S 'PLAYMOBIL' FIGURES AND DINGHY

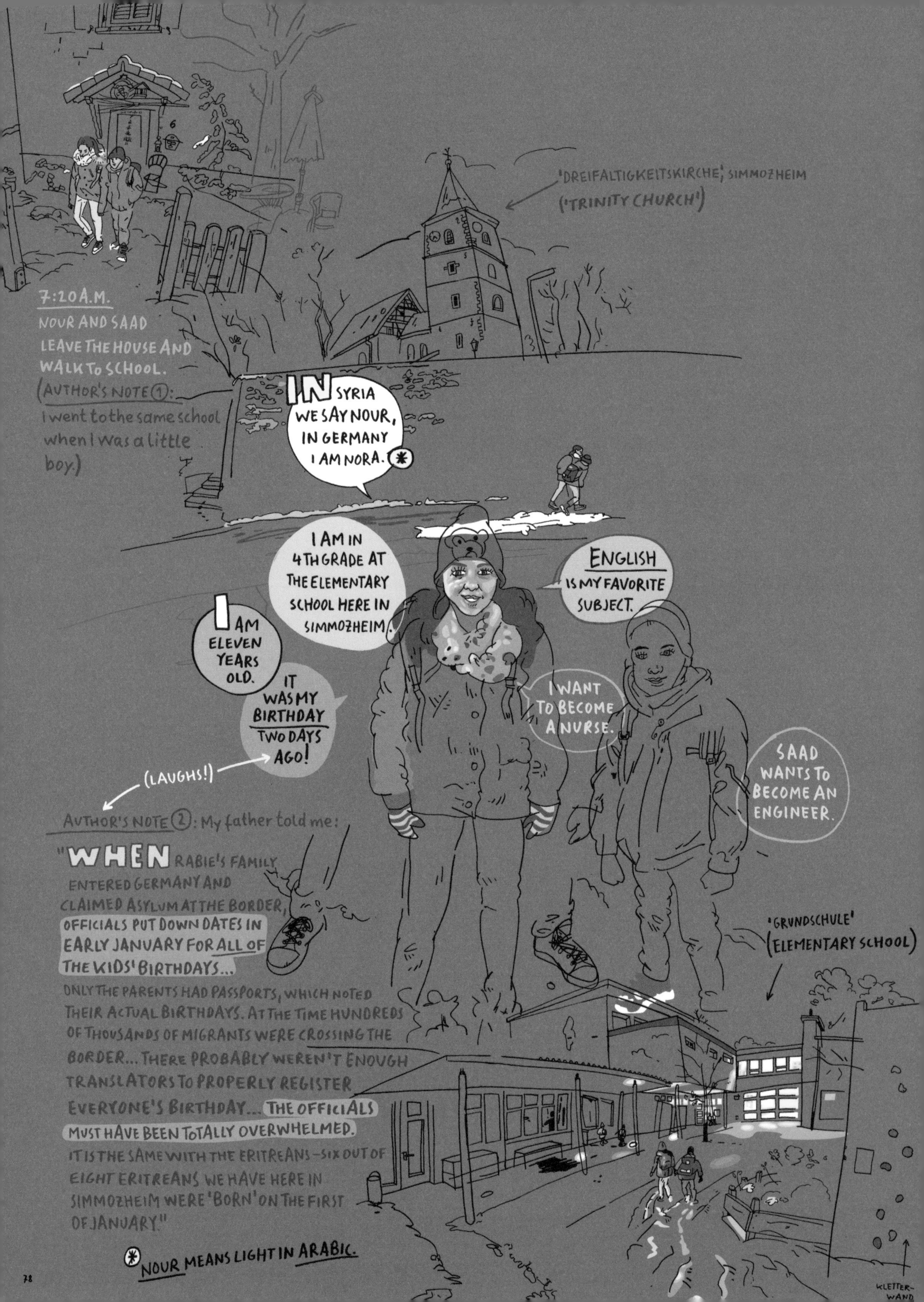

'DREIFALTIGKEITSKIRCHE,' SIMMOZHEIM ('TRINITY CHURCH')
7:20 A.M.
NOUR AND SAAD LEAVE THE HOUSE AND WALK TO SCHOOL.
(AUTHOR'S NOTE ①: I went to the same school when I was a little boy.)
IN SYRIA WE SAY NOUR, IN GERMANY I AM NORA. ✱
I AM IN 4TH GRADE AT THE ELEMENTARY SCHOOL HERE IN SIMMOZHEIM.
ENGLISH IS MY FAVORITE SUBJECT.
I AM ELEVEN YEARS OLD.
IT WAS MY BIRTHDAY TWO DAYS AGO!
I WANT TO BECOME A NURSE.
SAAD WANTS TO BECOME AN ENGINEER.
(LAUGHS!)
AUTHOR'S NOTE ②: My father told me:
"WHEN RABIE'S FAMILY ENTERED GERMANY AND CLAIMED ASYLUM AT THE BORDER, OFFICIALS PUT DOWN DATES IN EARLY JANUARY FOR ALL OF THE KIDS' BIRTHDAYS...
ONLY THE PARENTS HAD PASSPORTS, WHICH NOTED THEIR ACTUAL BIRTHDAYS. AT THE TIME HUNDREDS OF THOUSANDS OF MIGRANTS WERE CROSSING THE BORDER... THERE PROBABLY WEREN'T ENOUGH TRANSLATORS TO PROPERLY REGISTER EVERYONE'S BIRTHDAY... THE OFFICIALS MUST HAVE BEEN TOTALLY OVERWHELMED.
IT IS THE SAME WITH THE ERITREANS—SIX OUT OF EIGHT ERITREANS WE HAVE HERE IN SIMMOZHEIM WERE 'BORN' ON THE FIRST OF JANUARY."
'GRUNDSCHULE' (ELEMENTARY SCHOOL)
✱ NOUR MEANS LIGHT IN ARABIC.
KLETTER-WAND

POSTSCRIPT:

In February 2016, during a short stay in Switzerland, I had the chance to meet Nihad, the former member of MSF's psychological team, who I met in Domiz two years previously. Niina Tanskanen, from MSF Zürich, joined me on this visit. She speaks Arabic.

In August 2015, Nihad and his wife Avin decided to leave the refugee camp with their little daughter Naz. The three of them started their exhausting and dangerous 21-day journey to Switzerland, via Turkey, Greece, Macedonia, Serbia, Hungary and Austria.

It was very nice to see Nihad again and to meet his small family. After a delicious Syrian lunch in their cozy flat, Nihad told me:

"I FELT VERY CLOSELY CONNECTED WITH MY PATIENTS IN DOMIZ AND I FOUND IT DIFFICULT TO LEAVE THEM. I OFTEN SUFFER FROM A BAD CONSCIENCE."

05.02.2016 WITTENBACH, CLOSE TO ST. GALLEN, SWITZERLAND.
IN THE LIVING ROOM.

NIHAD
IS WORRIED ABOUT HIS MOTHER. SHE IS STILL IN QAMISHLI.
(*)
CAT IN GERMAN →
KATZE!
EINS, ZWEI, DREI...
← SHE CAN ALREADY COUNT TO TEN IN GERMAN.
AVIN, 23 YEARS OLD, STUDIED ECONOMICS IN ALEPPO.
NAZ, SHE HAD HER THIRD BIRTHDAY LAST WEEK.
PRINCESS-DRESS (A BIRTHDAY PRESENT)

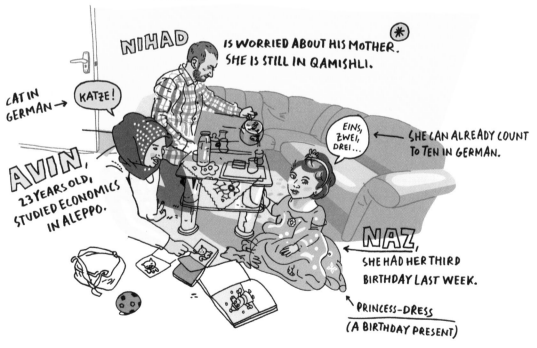

(*) Nihad's sick mother was granted a humanitarian visa to join them six months later, in the summer of 2016. Since then, she has lived with them.

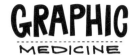

Susan Merrill Squier and Ian Williams, General Editors

Editorial Collective

MK Czerwiec (Northwestern University)

Michael J. Green (Penn State University College of Medicine)

Kimberly R. Myers (Penn State University College of Medicine)

Scott T. Smith (Penn State University)

Books in the Graphic Medicine series are inspired by a growing awareness of the value of comics as an important resource for communicating about a range of issues broadly termed "medical." For healthcare practitioners, patients, families, and caregivers dealing with illness and disability, graphic narrative enlightens complicated or difficult experience. For scholars in literary, cultural, and comics studies, the genre articulates a complex and powerful analysis of illness, medicine, and disability and a rethinking of the boundaries of "health." The series includes original comics from artists and non-artists alike, such as self-reflective "graphic pathographies" or comics used in medical training and education, as well as monographic studies and edited collections from scholars, practitioners, and medical educators.

Other titles in the series:

MK Czerwiec, Ian Williams, Susan Merrill Squier, Michael J. Green, Kimberly R. Myers, and Scott T. Smith, *Graphic Medicine Manifesto*

Ian Williams, *The Bad Doctor: The Troubled Life and Times of Dr. Iwan James*

Peter Dunlap-Shohl, *My Degeneration: A Journey Through Parkinson's*

Aneurin Wright, *Things to Do in a Retirement Home Trailer Park: . . . When You're 29 and Unemployed*

Dana Walrath, *Aliceheimers: Alzheimer's Through the Looking Glass*

Lorenzo Servitje and Sherryl Vint, eds., *The Walking Med: Zombies and the Medical Image*

Henny Beaumont, *Hole in the Heart: Bringing Up Beth*

MK Czerwiec, *Taking Turns: Stories from HIV/AIDS Care Unit 371*

Paula Knight, *The Facts of Life*

Gareth Brookes, *A Thousand Coloured Castles*

Jenell Johnson, ed., *Graphic Reproduction: A Comics Anthology*

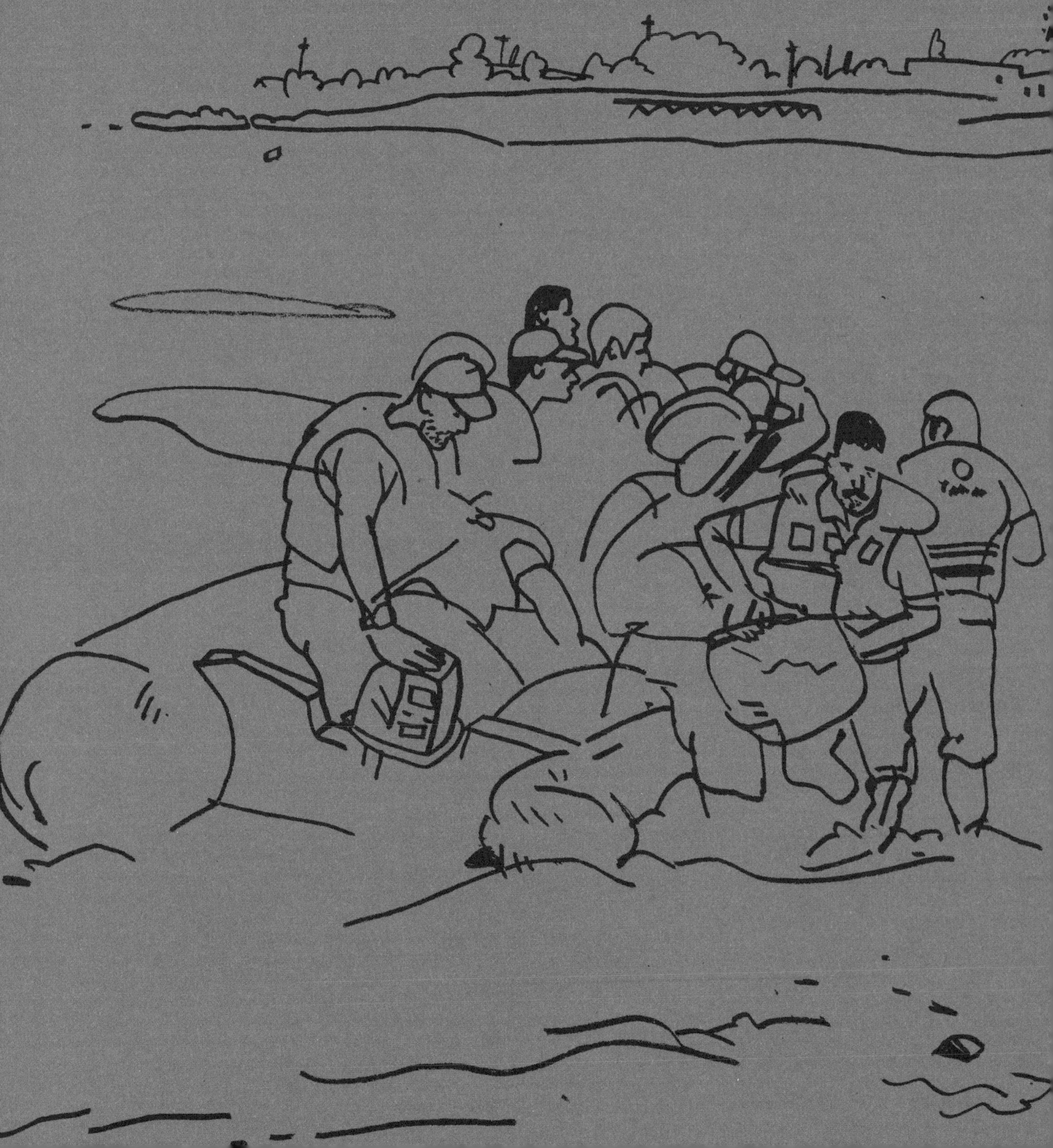